FACES OF POF

LEARNING AND LIVING WITH

PREMATURE OVARIAN FAILURE

COMPILED BY

THE PREMATURE OVARIAN FAILURE SUPPORT GROUP

FOREWORD BY NANETTE SANTORO, M.D.

FACES of POF

LEARNING AND LIVING WITH PREMATURE OVARIAN FAILURE

Copyright © 2004 by
The International Premature Ovarian Failure Support Group, Inc.

Published by
The International Premature Ovarian Failure Support Group, Inc.

Printed in the United States of America

ISBN: 1-931947-12-0

Library of Congress Card Number 2003097627

DEDICATION

This book is dedicated to all who contributed their stories to this book. Your generous sharing has blessed our lives and will, we know, bless the lives of all who read them.

AUTHORS' NOTE

The Premature Ovarian Failure Support Group (POFSG) is a non-profit organization whose mission is to provide community, support, and information to women with Premature Ovarian Failure (POF) and their loved ones; to increase public awareness and understanding of POF; and to work with health care professionals to better understand this condition. We are governed by an eight-member board and are independent of vested interests. Stories published reflect the experience and opinions of the writers. This book does not attempt to replace your health care provider. It does not constitute the practice of medicine. All matters regarding health require medical supervision.

Reading this book assumes that you have read this note. If you do not wish to be bound by the above, you may return this book to the publisher for a full refund.

FOREWORD

This is a book about hope. It is a book about survival. You will not find helpless victims inside these pages. You will become acquainted with a series of strong women, the men who love them, and their families. You will learn how individuals cope successfully with the adversity of this very challenging condition.

Premature ovarian failure is, by all accounts, a devastating diagnosis. Peculiar symptoms often last for years before a correct diagnosis is made. Women with this disorder may not attribute their symptoms to menopause—why would they? Their health care providers also tend to misattribute symptomatology. Diagnostic testing is delayed, sometimes resulting in irreversible loss of bone density and premature osteoporosis. And the often irreversible and unexpected infertility that accompanies POF is frequently the most distressing blow.

How do women adapt to this unwelcome diagnosis? In my years of experience in providing medical care to women with POF, there are some common themes that emerge. One of the most powerful affirmations for women with this diagnosis is the knowledge that they are not alone and that they can help one another. The Internet has become a true information highway for women with POF. By uniting those with a relatively rare disorder, sharing of emotions as well as medical knowledge can provide much support. POFers can help each other find the doctors who will work with them, the hormones (or alternatives) that will keep their symptoms at bay and their bodies healthy, and the wherewithal to wait it out until some of the answers they need come to them.

In this way, POF victims can make the transition into POF survivors.

In this book, you will find suggestions and hope that will help guide you or a loved one through this difficult diagnosis. There is no one answer for the infertility that so often accompanies POF: from adoption, to child-free living, to egg donation; the reader can try on each solution and see how it fits. Learning how to live with uncertainty is one of the central life lessons that POF forces women to acknowledge. Adaptation is an ongoing process that entails great personal growth, and this book will help to show you how to begin.

Nanette Santoro, M.D.
Professor and Director,
Division of Reproductive Endocrinology
Albert Einstein College of Medicine
Montefiore Medical Center

ACKNOWLEDGMENTS

Without the support we received, this book could not have been created. The biggest debt of thanks goes to the women, husbands, mothers and sisters who opened their hearts and lives to share their stories with you. Without them this book would not have been possible.

We are grateful for the many hands that made this book possible. The POFSG wishes to thank:

The POFSG board: Lisa Branick, Cori Canty Woessner, Suzanne Graf, Mary Jessup, Trinita McCall and Kelly Sigro. Without your absolute trust in this project it would not have been possible.

Drs. Nanette Santoro and Lawrence Nelson. You have both been invaluable to the POF community and you continue to give of yourselves. We are humbled by your presence here.

Melody Graham, Christine Sanchez, Carmen Simpson and Beth Wilkie for your sharp eyes, insights and for reading through the many stories to find the best ones to share with our readers.

Susan M. Raaths, Jennifer's mother and an English teacher, who dedicated her time to reading, correcting and commenting on the final story selections.

The Endocrine Nurses Society. Without their startup grant, this project would not have begun. Thank you for your faith in our organization.

Jackie Bogert (former POFSG board member and book coordinator) who caught the vision with such enthusiasm and camaraderie. Thanks for listening for hours, at all hours, to share the vision.

Mike Bjarko, our editor, we couldn't have done this without your encouragement and direction.

Marlo Schalesky and Chris and Pat Sheffield who shared their insights on the monumental writing tasks we'd all undertaken and for their encouragement to pursue the dream.

Sara Mcyers, for the generosity of your computer skills after our computer crashed.

Nicole Damberg, Amy Daniels, Tonya Lane, Michelle Mahenski, Sarah Poindexter, Rachel, Amy Utzig and Beth Wilkie. The definitions and resources dream team!

This book came together with a degree of creative ingenuity that we only dreamed of. This is due to the immense talents and contributions of: James Taylor, cover photographer; Debbie Struiksma who had the inspiration to take a photo of young women with POF; the POFers who allowed their photos be taken; E.M.C., cover design; Amy Selby who came up with a title that was a universal hit; and Mike Bjarko for the book's interior layout and design.

Jennifer Raaths, who generously gave of her time, talent and expertise in this compilation. She encouraged and nurtured women to contribute stories, edited stories and arranged the story order. This project wouldn't have come to fruition without her.

From Jennifer; Thank you to my husband Dan and son Alex for giving me the time and support to work on this project.

From Catherine; To Donald, your humor and tenderness are central to my life. I could not have devoted the time to this project without your patience.

One last group—It's not easy to be a good friend when something like POF happens. Thank you to all the friends and family who care, through thick and thin, and help keep us together. You know who you are and you're loved.

Proceeds of this book help to support educational programs of the POFSG.

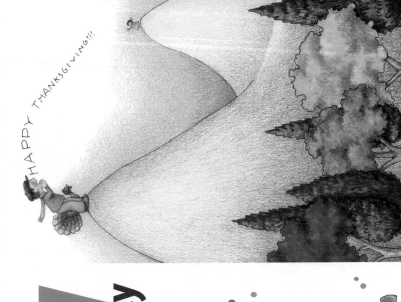

HAPPY THANKSGIVING!!!

nov
thursday
24

Thanksgiving (USA)

Josette Degiorgio

POf support

Group

Jdegiorgio@hotmail.com

Having Your Baby Through
55 Dunston
Glazer

CONTENTS

Contents (cont.)

INTRODUCTION

"Stories seem to awaken new energies of love; they tell us great truths in simple, personal terms and make us long for light. Stories have a strange power of attraction. When we tell stories, we touch hearts...

...When we hear stories of others who have lived as we live and how they have risen up from the drab and found hope, we, too, find hope."

—Jean Vanier, *Becoming Human*, 1998, pages 90-91

The value of community is central to most of us. The belief that those with POF are sustained by a community is at the core of this book. The POF community is one in which the sharing of our stories is vital to healing and growing. We have been blessed by a community rich with those who teach us through the stories you are going to read. Safe in each other's hands, we can be open and vulnerable to one another. The deeper I went into my soul, listened to the stories of others and shared my story, I received a generosity of spirit that helped my own healing.

This book is about healing. It is about discovering our path and carefully walking it with the help and blessing of the community of people within these covers. It started with our own journeys. It resonates with our own experiences of trying to make sense of our diagnoses and struggles in trying to understand why we had this trial. Few, besides those experiencing POF, deal with something like this. Within the POF community we can find understanding. Feeling alone, we hoped that a book of stories would bring comfort not only to us but to other women as well. As stories were shared we encountered a type of wisdom and comfort we hadn't found in the reams of material on infertility or menopause. Friends have no experience comparable to this and are sometimes puzzled by our changing moods, inability to attend baby showers, talk of no sleep, unexplained aches and pains and hot flashes.

This book is the work of women and their families who have been through the heartache and confusion that are often linked with a diagnosis of POF. They are reaching out a hand to those who are now experiencing the same pain they had. They know what it means to experience a POF diagnosis. You'll see that most have also learned how to pick up and continue on their life's journey and they share some of their hard-earned wisdom with you. In your POF journey you may recognize yourself in the authors of some of these stories and you may find comfort knowing that you are not alone.

Many women reading this book won't know that what they are experiencing are the normal stages of grief. That is what women with POF experience: a death—loss of dreams, hopes, and plans. Five stages of grief have been identified: denial, anger, bargaining, depression and acceptance. The denial stage is characterized by feelings of numbness and isolation. We refuse to believe what has happened. We may keep vigilantly busy so that we don't have to focus on POF. The anger stage is often directed against our doctor, significant other or God. In bargaining, we often offer something to try to take away the reality of the diagnosis. We may try to make a deal, with ourselves or, if we are religious, with God. Depression is generally the most difficult stage to deal with. Feelings of listlessness and fatigue can be followed by bouts of intense emotion and tears. The final stage is acceptance. This is not synonymous with happiness. It is more an ability to make peace with our situation. It represents a time in which we begin to integrate our losses and to move to a newly defined life. We may not experience all these stages, or go through them in the same order, and we may reencounter them. What we experience is normal. Knowing that others have experienced the same feelings can bring some comfort.

None of us would have picked this for our lives. This isn't what we had planned. We would not have set out to become contributors to a book on POF. But this is the life we were given. We can spend our lives yearning for what might have been or we can let our "new" life be our teacher and allow this path that yields wisdom and understanding to be a time for growth.

From somewhere, people have the ability to endure losses and to start over again. For me, it is one of the great proofs of the existence of God. In this book you will read about women who rail against God, then ask Him into their lives again. To pick up from a POF diagnosis requires courage and resiliency and for me, the help of God. When the women recorded here began to heal, they often came back to their lives with a deeper, more mature, and wiser look on life.

The harsh fact of a diagnosis such as POF is that it may be an opportunity for fresh insight into our lives. We must take responsibility for new directions. It will help in our healing and hopefully to an even richer life. We must experience our losses fully and let the feelings surface. I hope you will be warmed by the light that envelopes you through this book of memory, anguish, coping and accepting.

Not every story has a happy ending. Not every storyteller has achieved acceptance. Some are depressed, addicted to alcohol or have renounced close relationships. The path continues for those storytellers.

This book can be read as a whole or as individual stories seen as separate stones on a walking path. It can be heart-lifting or heavy. Either way it will be a worthwhile endeavor. There are stories from around the world. We have tried to keep the voices of the authors unaltered. POF is an issue everywhere and reflected in the stories. Come back to this book and take from it what you need when you need it.

We have not sought the miraculous in this book. We can't erase POF. This is a book of the heart. By walking the path with you we hope you will find comfort here.

Catherine Corp
POFSG President
Director of Education and Research

PROLOGUE

Gifts from Young Women with Premature Ovarian Failure

Over the years, as a physician and as a research scientist, I have had the privilege of meeting many wonderful and courageous young women with premature ovarian failure. Each and every one of them have given me the opportunity to enter a very precious and tender area of their life. In doing so they have each given me a wonderful gift.

After all these years, I realize that these young women have changed my life. They have given me profound gifts. They have strengthened my faith in God. They have strengthened my faith in science. They have strengthened my understanding of religion and science as a marriage of faith and reason. They have taught me that hope, comfort, and spiritual strength are as important in maintaining our physical health as they are in maintaining our emotional health.

Catherine Corp, the founder of the Premature Ovarian Failure Support Group, has changed the landscape for many young women with premature ovarian failure by providing them comfort and inspiration. As a gynecologist conducting research on premature ovarian failure, I know personally how valuable her efforts have been to these young women. Winston Churchill was right; "We make a living by what we get, but we make a life by what we give." By that standard Catherine Corp is having a great life.

—Lawrence M. Nelson, M.D.

CHANGE OF LIFE

Lisa, thirty-seven, diagnosed at thirty-four

I was in my kitchen making a big batch of fried chicken while my two children, Matthew, five, and two-year-old Samantha, sat coloring at the table when the phone rang. It was my Ob/Gyn's associate, as my doctor was on vacation. I knew what she was calling about; my test results. I had been having problems with my cycle. I hadn't had my period for four months, and before that it had been very strange: either coming every couple of weeks or lapsing altogether. More troubling were the hot flashes and night sweats I was suffering. For months I had been having up to 100 intense hot flashes a day and was waking up several times a night drenched in sweat. What in the world could they be from? I had no clue.

The doctor said, "Lisa, I have your test results here, and it seems you are postmenopausal. How old are you again?"

I gulped as my heart reached my throat. "Thirty-four. I, um, just turned thirty-four," I said, as another hot flash suddenly raced through me.

"Oh yes, thirty-four. Well, you had better make an appointment to come in and get some estrogen. This is not good for someone your age."

"Okay," I stammered, and sensed she was about to hang up. "Wait! Why would this happen? Is it temporary? I was waiting for my period to come so I could try fertility drugs again to get pregnant. Can I still do that?"

She paused for a second and said, "It may be temporary, but it seems

3

unlikely. Your FSH level was sixty-nine and estrogen level less than ten, so you are postmenopausal now. I don't know about getting pregnant again. You would have to talk to a fertility specialist about that. Make an appointment and we'll discuss hormone replacement therapy for you."

My hand started to shake as I hung up the phone. I am in MENOPAUSE? I felt sick to my stomach. I took the chicken off the stove and threw it in the trash. I ran in to my bathroom, being careful to close the door so my kids could not hear me crying. The room spun as I hung my head over the toilet and threw up. I called my husband at work and tried to tell him between sobs what the doctor had said. He said he would come home as soon as he could, and I tried to pull myself together so my kids would not see me in such a state.

By the time my husband got home I was seesawing between thinking this just had to be some big mistake and knowing in my heart that this is why I had been feeling so badly for months. I had recently noticed many changes in my body. My hair and skin felt dry and looked "different" to me when I looked in the mirror. I had gained about seven pounds, and instead of ending up around my hips and thighs like usual, it had all accumulated around my middle like my husband's "love handles." I had noticed that I was dry everywhere; my eyes, my mouth, and most of all my vaginal area. It had become very painful to make love to my husband.

My husband also had a hard time believing it, so I made an appointment to see a specialist as well as my doctor. This had to be just a strange reaction to weaning my two-year-old daughter, which I had done a few months earlier in order to start fertility treatments for our third child. We were able to conceive our first two after much heartache and trying with the combination of Clomid and progesterone. This had to work again. I had to have another child.

A few weeks later I sat in my doctor's office full of anticipation. I tried to act upbeat and downplayed my hot flashes and night sweats, so that she would think this was some kind of mistake, too. She gave me a lab slip for another blood test, and when I asked about getting pregnant she said, "I'm recommending you see a reproductive endocrinologist." She gave me a referral slip for that, too. "I'll bet there is still time to help you get pregnant!" I left with so much hope. We did not talk about HRT at this appointment because I felt there was no reason to.

A few days later I got a message on my answering machine. My results were the same as before, postmenopausal. I was heartbroken, and felt so alone. Had anyone ever gone through menopause at this age? Never were the words "premature ovarian failure" used. I only learned about this much later when I was researching in the library. I clung to the hope that the fertility doctor would be able to help me, and figured at least I would be able to get pregnant one more time before menopause.

The RE led me to his office and sat across from me at his desk. I was surprised that he did not need to examine me. He said he had read my file, and asked how could he help me. I explained my fertility history, how I had gotten pregnant twice with the help of fertility drugs, and was willing to go for the "big guns" this time to make it happen.

He cleared his throat and said, "Well, unfortunately what you have is ovarian failure, so any fertility drug that we have would not help you."

I kept interrupting him, asking, "Can't we just try Pergonal, or some other injectable…" but he kept saying firmly, "No, it just won't work. But we do have another option called egg donation. That is where we take eggs from another woman, fertilize them with your husband's sperm and implant them in you. You would be a wonderful candidate for this because you have successfully carried two children to term already."

I knew a little about egg donation, because I had read that it may be my only option, but it seemed so strange to me at the time. I said "I don't know, we did talk about adopting a baby girl from China."

He responded, "You could do that, but you don't know what you are getting—no information on the birthparents, or prenatal care. You take

5

away that risk with egg donation."

My head was spinning. I drove home in a daze and told my husband in hushed tones (so the kids would not hear) what the doctor had said. He held me and we cried together. He said he would be willing to look into both egg donation and adoption and we would decide together what was the best choice.

In the meantime I had not started HRT yet, and felt terrible. I was hot-flashing all day and night, waking up two times a night just to change my nightgown that would get soaked through with sweat. I felt so old and undesirable. It made me sick to think about being in menopause. I made an appointment to see a doctor about HRT and she also examined me. She commented that my vagina looked "pretty atrophied" and handed me my prescription. She said to take estrogen on days one to twenty-five and progesterone on days twelve to twenty-five. I thought that she meant to take it on the first day of my cycle, which had not shown itself at that point, but she actually meant to take it on the first day of the month.

It now seems silly that I made this mistake, but I was so misinformed about my condition, and had no clue about what was going on with my body. I did not even know that it was unlikely my period would ever come back. I waited for months, suffering with the hot flashes and, even worse, the depression. I felt like the happiness part of my brain was switched off.

I finally called her, told her how depressed I was feeling, and could I please start my HRT even though it was not "Day 1." She seemed perplexed, but said, "It will mess up your days, but go ahead." She never asked me about the depression.

I started my HRT and did feel better. At least the hot flashes slowed down and I felt more like my old self as far as my moods. I got the results of my bone density test that I had asked for (and was told I did not need) and discovered I had osteopenia of the neck, hip and almost osteoporosis in the spine. I looked into different calcium supplements and went to the drugstore to get some information about bone loss and menopause. All the brochures had pictures of old women playing tennis with slogans like, "Life can still be good after fifty!" I felt like there was no one I could talk to about this who could understand. My friends were clueless about what this meant for me and seemed to think it was no big deal. I even had one say, "You are lucky, you're all done with menopause!" I did have one good friend who cried with me over my diagnosis and tried to understand.

We still had our hearts and minds on our third child. So we made appointments with an international adoption agency and an egg donation clinic. Although the idea of egg donation no longer seemed so strange, we both felt pulled toward adopting a baby girl from China. When I closed my eyes I could see her face and I felt a happiness I had not felt in a long time. So we signed all the paperwork and started the laborious process of paperwork and home studies.

Around this time I ventured online for the first time in my life. I found the Websites www.EarlyMenopause.com and the POF support board, www.PofSupport.org. There were actually other women like me—young and in menopause! I posted my story on the POFer to POFer board and was amazed and thrilled by the support and understanding I received from these women whom I did not know. It became my lifeline and I still visit the board every day.

All the women there were my biggest supporters in our adoption journey. When I met my husband at the airport with our new daughter Emma Juliet, I could not wait to rush home and tell all my POFer friends about it.

I also gained great information there, especially about different kinds of HRTs. I finally found a combination that works well for me (Estrace and Prometrium) and I feel great now. I admit I don't feel the same as I did before this happened; I feel "changed" in a very profound way. But I have learned in the past two years that life can be good and sweet and wonderful after a diagnosis of premature ovarian failure.

DO I HAVE REGRETS?

Lorain, fifty-one, diagnosed at thirty-one

When I was diagnosed at the age of thirty-one in 1983, having had symptoms for four years, I was told it was premature menopause. I never even heard the term premature ovarian failure until sometime in 2001, when I was poking around the Internet and stumbled across it. I found the term on a site for rare disorders. To this day, my younger sister (who was fully menopausal by her early forties) is the only other person I know who had begun menopause before the "normal" age. I have felt for two decades like a true oddity among women. I know other women who are coping with the sadness of not being able to have children—caused by endometriosis, early hysterectomy, and so forth—but none with POF.

I am quite sure that my POF was genetically caused. According to my mother, my paternal grandmother told her that she never had a period after her youngest child, my aunt, was born when she was thirty-eight. I take after my paternal grandmother more than any of her other grandchildren, and have always been glad of it—until this! Additionally, since my younger sister also was early, we conjecture that the disposition for the POF might have been handed down through our father. We decided a couple of years ago to tell the next generation in our family. We have four teen-aged nieces, born within six years of each other: two daughters of our older sister, whose menopause has been at a "normal" age, and two daughters of our older brother.

With the work done on the Human Genome Project in these last

9

several years, there has been shown to be a gene that can mutate and thereby cause POF. I did see an endocrinologist after my diagnosis because there was some concern that if my ovaries had shut down, other glands might also have done so, thus presenting a much greater systemic concern. Fortunately, that was not so. Part of that work-up involved some genetic evaluation, but there simply was not the technology back then that there is now.

At the time, I also wondered if my POF was related to the fact that my mother took DES when she was pregnant with me. I was born in 1951, when DES was still being prescribed by doctors in Boston. Every doctor that she or I have ever talked to has insisted that there is absolutely no connection. I have no reason not to believe that, especially since my older sister, born in 1950 and menopausal at a "normal age," is also a DES daughter. Also, my younger sister, early menopausal, is not a DES daughter; by 1955, when she was born, doctors were no longer prescribing DES because its dangers were already becoming apparent.

For a long time I thought the POF was entirely stress-triggered: within three years in my late twenties, I was separated and divorced, my mother contracted colon cancer, I remarried and gained two young stepchildren, and a very dear friend died of brain cancer. I was diagnosed with POF soon after all of this. For many years I agonized over how I could have handled that stretch of time—and all that stress—differently, so as to have put my body on a different physiological and hormonal path. It was a tremendous relief, beyond words, to know that there probably is a genetic cause that I simply inherited, and that nothing I could have done, from the day I was conceived, would have changed the fact that at thirty-one I would be menopausal.

After my diagnosis in 1983, my husband and I did investigate our options. Both my sisters offered eggs, which was just incredible. I was told by my infertility specialist that my menopausal body could not support and bring to term a pregnancy, even with a "good egg." My younger sister even offered to bear a child for me, by artificial insemination using my husband's sperm. She was single at the time, so that would have been quite a gift, and, technically, it would have been surrogate motherhood. Even if I had been able successfully to pursue pregnancy with an egg from one of my sisters, this was, remember, the early 1980s, still in the early days of our society sorting out the legal and bioethical issues of surrogate motherhood. In this case I, not my sister, would have been the surrogate mother, carrying her fertilized egg to term. There were only a couple places in New England, where I live, that were even venturing into that legal and ethical territory at that point in time.

I also was not prepared to predict the heavy-laden emotional consequences far enough into the future to know how using a sister's egg, or having a sister bear a child for me, would have totally transformed the dynamic in my family of origin for the rest of our lives. Finally, after all of these considerations, and also wrestling with my deep love for my two stepchildren—whom I was helping to raise, and yet looking into their faces, my heart would always break, for I couldn't see my own genetic history—we decided to stop all of the searching for options, including adoption. The emotional pingpong was becoming too much to bear.

Only a year or so after this did I begin to realize that the depth of my grief, which seemed at times unbearable, was the grief of losing a child—to be sure, a yet-to-be-conceived child. I could picture this child: it had the good looks of its father and the intelligence of its mother! I had names picked out. Still today, some twenty years later, I imagine this child as a young adult, in college, heading out into the world. The grief continues to wash over me.

When we moved from Massachusetts to Maine in 1993, I looked for a gynecologist who specialized in infertility. During my first visit that year, she asked me if I wanted to become pregnant. I could not believe my ears: I was forty-two at the time. She told me that doctors in Italy were doing some good work in enabling menopausal women to carry pregnancies to term. I surprised myself at how quickly I said no. Too many lives, not the least of which was my own, would have been disrupted at that point. I realized then that I had moved forward in my journey with this reality of my life, since, for a number of years early on, I would have literally sold my soul in order to bear a child.

Do I have regrets? A few. I am not sure I would have made the same decisions now knowing what I feel at fifty-one. I might have pursued adoption. But I also know that such life-transforming decisions are not made quickly. I was thirty-one when I was diagnosed, but my husband was already forty, and I felt that time was not on our side. Rather than being nagged by regret forever, I choose to honor the sadness instead. My life is full to the brim, and I have been able to pursue a different path than I might have had I raised my own children from birth.

At some point I also realized I had to let go of the "What if's," and "What would have happened if I had lived my life differently?" For example, when I was married the first time in my early twenties, I could have had a child. Do I regret not doing that now? Not one iota. It is difficult enough to live with the reality of POF, without taking on more anguish by wishing I had made different decisions.

But not for a moment does my moving on in my life's journey fill the emptiness. Nor does it erase the sense I have that there is a vast injustice in the universe.

The Donut

Anita, thirty-one, diagnosed at thirty

Goals are dreams with deadlines. So what happens when those dreams are shattered? Sitting in the gynaecology waiting room of our local hospital, surrounded by pregnant women, I smiled as I thought about how my life was progressing. With a career established, the big O.E. (overseas experience) now a distant memory, and an almost freehold house, it was now time to fulfill the next goal of starting a family. My partner of twelve years and I had just announced our intended marriage and I had been referred to the hospital by my doctor to organise medication to "kick-start" my menstrual cycle and try for a baby. Everything was going as planned. Nothing could have prepared me for what I was about to be told.

Me? Premature menopause? I had just turned thirty, with what ended up being my last period ten months earlier. The gynaecologist said to me, "You seem to be taking this okay—are you alright?" I thought, "Why me?" but I already knew the answer—"Why not?" Looking back now, I guess I was in shock. I just sat there, numb.

The gynaecologist bundled me up with all sorts of reading material about menopause. He had even arranged for me to see the fertility clinic that same day.

The nurse at the fertility clinic explained IVF briefly to me, although I can't say I really took much in at the time. She gave me some examples of advertisements in the paper for donors and kindly stated that *Little Treasures* and *Next* magazines were the best. The nurse then asked if I'd like our names put on the waiting list. I told her I'd found out only two hours earlier and would actually like to discuss it with my fiancé first!

When I got home I opened up one of the books on menopause and began reading: "For some women it's a time of relief that contraceptive measures are no longer needed, a time to enjoy your interests and spend time with your grandchildren."…and later… "After all, after menopause you still have one-third of your life left."

Well that was the end of the reading material for me! I felt like I had a young spirit trapped inside an old body. I felt cheated.

All of a sudden I wasn't in the driver's seat anymore. I was out of control and going somewhere I never planned to go. The worst part for me was the realisation that I would NEVER be able to reproduce myself—"us." Having no sisters meant that I would need to get donor eggs from someone else. That's been the hardest to accept. For weeks I told no one. My fiancé and I started discussing the options of waiting for a donor or asking a friend. It got more complicated the more we thought about all of the implications. I didn't feel comfortable asking a friend because I thought about how I'd feel being asked myself.

Telling my mum was the hardest. I really felt like I'd failed her, so when I talked to her I tried to act as if it wasn't such a big deal. The thing was, she felt worse because she felt she'd failed me!

It's difficult to decide whom to tell. All the time you have people making comments such as, "It's your turn next." Sometimes I've wanted to turn and tell them I can't have children, just to see the look on their faces. Then again, it's not their fault. It's a natural assumption that I've even been guilty of myself.

It's been five months now since I was diagnosed. Since then we've had our wedding and I'm finding I'm telling a few more people along the way. I guess it's part of the process of accepting what has happened. I'm also part of a study to try to detect early menopause.

On the lighter side:

- I don't have to worry about contraception anymore
- My husband will never need to have a vasectomy
- I definitely didn't have mad cow disease last year when I thought I was going mad!

We've just found out that we have been accepted for one free IVF cycle through the hospital and a friend has offered to be a donor. So, fingers crossed for the end of the year, but if it's not meant to be I guess our next question will be, "What's in God's OTHER hand?" Meanwhile it's full steam ahead with the rest of our lives. Although there may be a void in my life, it's so important to look at the donut and not the hole.

Eaglewoman Sings

Fiona, thirty-one, diagnosed at twenty-nine

I ran excitedly through wavy pastures, following long flowing skirts, brushing through shawls as I snuggled into a circle of women who waited, laughing, timeless in the August sun.

Manati, a Taino-Arawak woman raised in the Bronx, called us closer with a hearty grin and a soft, gentle strength, "Come, come, make room for everyone." The fringes of her shawl danced as she spoke. She told us about the origins and meanings of the traditional moon time teachings. I pondered the beauty of twenty-eight days, revolving season after season, tides beckoning their weight to the moonlit nights, bodies rising, turning, women letting their bloods flow into the heart of the earth, gathered women weaving stories saying, "This is how it was for me." One by one, they shared as women, in the space we had created. I listened to one, two, three, then wondered, "Where am I in this?"

As quickly as it had begun, the romance was broken. I scowled at the moon. Some high flung, neon lifesaver you turned out to be, I thought. Looking at the faces of my sisters I longed for any sign of recognition. They smiled back warmly, too warmly. I wanted to run.

My heart started racing...I don't belong here...I feel like an impostor, like a man sitting here listening to all you women sharing stories of your moon time. I'm thinking all this in my head and the beating gets so loud it's drowning out my thoughts. Before I know it I'm speaking out loud, telling these women I met only days ago that I haven't bled in two years. I'm twenty-eight and that last time it was just once that whole year. It'd been on and off for years before that. No one can tell me what's going on. I'm stressed, my heart is pounding.

I see a shawl sweep across the center of the circle, "Come child, come." Like an eagle wing she beckons me. I hear drumming. Is it in my heart or is it outside of me? I'm scared, but I stand and allow her to wrap her wings around me. Manati stands beside us. Circling, Eaglewoman tells me my blood has all dried up. "You have given all you have to give to the earth. Now you must give to a wider family. The grandmothers are calling you. You must give to many people."

This is too much for me to hear. I cry huge sobs. Inside everything revolts. As much as I never got tired of not having my moon, I wasn't ready to have it taken. How can the grandmothers call me when I'm twenty-eight? Why me? No, I think, I don't want this to be. Manati's grandchildren sit sprawled on a blanket giggling corn ear smiles, shaking their rattles; the little one is humming to herself. I am shaken to my core. Manati throws a quick glance at the little one. "And so it's true," she says, "The little one is telling you."

The circle ends, a rush of green returns, the flattened grasses spring. One by one a sea of women grab me, hug me. They are moved and joyous. "What an honor to witness this," they say. Me, I am just in shock.

I am told to prepare a ceremony when I go back to Montreal, bring my friends together and celebrate this transition. It is a new beginning, being called to give in a new way.

I decided to go back and see more doctors first. A month later, they confirm premature ovarian failure. In the cold hospital walls, in the smallest windowless room, a resident gives me the news. The doctor doesn't have time to see me. I insist. He finally shows up, barely, just a head in a door behind me. "What does this mean, please tell me."

He sighs impatiently, he is angry. He writes a referral, telling me to call there for more information. Flippantly, as an afterthought once he's left the room, he turns back and says, "Oh, by the way, you have about one percent chance of ever having children."

18

I am left alone. Stunned. Spinning, the room becomes unreal. A few seconds later he returns, head in the doorway again, "Actually, no, no chance really." Then he's gone.

I scream obscenities at him in my head. I am left to wonder if he would have treated a white woman this way. I think, "Has he just read my chart? Is this homophobia? Does he think just because I don't sleep with men I don't care about being a mother?" I get so tired of having to wonder, but never tired enough to not feel the rage.

I don't remember what the resident looked like or how she got me out of that seat, but I will never forget that doctor's face. The inhumanity of that moment, that very precious moment.

I couldn't risk driving home. The car stayed in the hospital's lot that day. I walked like I have never walked before in my life—steaming, fast. I barely put the key in the lock before yelling into the empty corners of my home. Pillows flew in all directions. I'm not a person to swear a lot, but that day I made up for all the time I never claimed. Luckily, I had a lot of swear words in the bank.

My referral was short-lived. He was an old flirt who told me that women used to die shortly after their childbearing years. He droned on and on about how women's bodies get progressively worse in the post-menopausal years. In other words, it was all downhill from here and nature dictated that woman's main role was to give birth, then die. Suddenly, the drumming, the rattles, the children's giggles and the teachings of the moon circle sounded really good.

Words of the past came back to me, strengthening me. I have something to give, to give to a wider family. My life, a new life, is just beginning, not ending.

I bid good riddance to him and set off to find a more inspiring doctor, one who would have a more positive view of women, one who would also understand the role of culture and traditions in healing. I fasted and decided that if I am going to take hormone replacement therapy, then I also want to follow other ways of healing as well. Over the

19

years I have experimented with jin shin do, traditional healing in the sweat lodge, diet, swimming, weight training, meditation, prayer, and dance in combination with HRT. It's a continuous journey, continuously learning.

As a young person, going into the hospitals and having tests which normally older people go through teaches me to be humble. When I see the older people waiting on stretchers, ravaged by chemotherapy, alone, and so ill, I remember to be kinder and gentler. I remember to be grateful for the health that I do have. Most of all, I remember how short our time here really is, and how strong and fragile all of us can be.

ECHO CHAMBER

Anne, thirty-seven, diagnosed at thirty

Unmoored
Unmourned
Unhinged at the Knees

Moonless

An old, old, young woman
shrunken with death
never swollen with life

Scooped out, hollowed
Hobbles her good-byes:
red shock, smell of spring dirt, life line, uterine tears,
tides, dreams, youth

The warm, safe future space
is an echo chamber

Listen:
    voices of past and future
    fading
    faded
    gone

FEARFULLY AND WONDERFULLY MADE

Rachel, forty-four, diagnosed at nineteen

I was born and raised in a small, isolated, northern Canadian community, the third of five children. I had a good childhood.

I started noticing that I was not like other girls when my teen years began. One by one, my girlfriends started their periods and began wearing bras, while my body remained childlike. Then my younger sister got her period and surpassed me in height by four inches. All the neighbours thought she was older than I.

My mother seemed somewhat unconcerned about my "stunted" growth, as she had not started menstruating until she was fifteen. I, on the other hand, felt very self-conscious and began feeling increasingly uncomfortable. Thankfully, most of my girlfriends were kind and never ridiculed me; yet I still yearned, with all my heart, to begin the process toward womanhood.

One day, I excitedly told my mother that I had finally noticed a little bleeding and that the time must have come at last. She then gave me a pad and belt (this was the seventies, before self-adhesive pads) and proceeded to show me how to wear this new "getup." I was so relieved. Now I was going to be like all the other girls my age. The relief was short-lived when I discovered that the bleeding was haemorrhoids of all things. Another letdown.

I first visited my family doctor about this problem at fourteen or fif-

23

teen. All I can remember about it was my devastation when he told me that I was never going to bear children. I ran home and told my mom. I was expecting sympathy and a hug from her. What I received instead was an expression of great relief for me that I would not have to suffer the pains of childbirth and all the trials that went with it. Even my mom didn't understand the deep pain I felt.

The summer of my sixteenth year, my parents felt that I should see a specialist. Off we went by train to a nearby city to see an obstetrician/gynaecologist (Ob/Gyn) for examination, diagnosis and hopefully a cure. My hopes were up. They were dashed again when, after his examination and questions, he informed us that tests and exploratory surgery could not take place until I was eighteen years old. That was definitely not what I had hoped to hear. I felt he had no idea what two whole years of waiting meant to someone my age. In my mind, I felt that by then my youth and a very important part of my social life as a "budding" adult would be over.

If the doctors couldn't help me, I was going to take things into my own hands. My options were limited at this point, but I resolved to appear as a young woman by the time school began that fall. This will sound funny, but I was desperate. I was through wearing baggy shirts that helped to conceal my flat chest. I was still wearing a training bra, though I had turned seventeen over the summer. I carefully padded it with tissues to a size that resembled my sister's size A chest. This worked fine and made my last two years of high school more bearable. To this day, I don't remember telling any of my close friends what I had done. I could never risk the word getting out. I would have been so embarrassed if it had.

In September 1978, the summer after my high school graduation, my doctor sent me to a Toronto hospital for five days of tests, x-rays and abdominal exploratory surgery. X-rays were taken of my head to see if there were any tumours on my pituitary gland that could have prevented normal puberty. At the end of the week of tests, my mom came up to Toronto and together we met with the Ob/Gyn. They had found that, though my uterus was normal, the ovaries had never developed. There was only a small amount of tissue where they should have been. As a result, my growth in height and normal puberty had never taken place. When I asked about child bearing, he said that the normal way was out of the question. He then put me on a contraceptive called Ovral. This, he explained, would give me a regular period and start normal breast development. At nineteen I was going to begin puberty.

Most of my friends had left for college or university by this time. It was too late for me to apply to go away to school so I looked for work instead and found a great job. I dated a few fellows during the next few years, but none of them seriously. After three years of working in my small community, I applied for a transfer to a nearby city. I got the job.

When I moved there, I found an Ob/Gyn who referred me to an endocrinologist. The endocrinologist took me off contraceptives and put me on estrogen and progesterone. I took estrogen from the first to the twenty-fifth of each month and progesterone from the sixteenth to the twenty-fifth. This most closely resembled the normal female cycle and still made it relatively easy to keep the dates straight. My breasts grew slightly more and my periods became a little heavier. I grew from five feet, two inches at nineteen to five feet five at twenty-three. I now matched my sisters in height. Later, the endocrinologist also advised me that I was to remain on these hormones indefinitely to prevent bone loss and osteoporosis. When I questioned him about the length of time, he explained that he never prescribed anything with a view beyond twenty years in the future.

The years went by as I led the life of a single lady in a city. Medically, there was nothing unusual, but in April 1988, I became anxious, was unable to concentrate at work, and I felt like crying for no reason. My family doctor diagnosed it as clinical depression. I couldn't account for it because until then I had always been a happy, optimistic person. My doctor also noticed that my cholesterol level was getting very high for someone in their late twenties. I've since discovered a possible link between hormone replacement therapy and a problem with the metabolism of fat in the body.

I am now forty-one and I've been on various doses of an antidepressant since April 1988. I've also had to miss a lot of work as a result. Neither my family doctor nor my endocrinologist would admit that the depression was in any way related to POF. I still have my doubts about that. I'm currently seeing a naturopathic physician who has given me vitamins and herbs that I hope will help over time.

I'm still unmarried and content with that. Nevertheless, I have not ruled out marriage and would welcome the "right" man should God send him my way. Now that I'm forty-one, the prospect of not bearing children is far less of an issue. Should it ever become an issue to a potential mate, I would welcome the idea of adoption with joy. For now, I enjoy being an auntie.

Finally, I must say that I could not be so lighthearted about my medical situation were it not for my strong belief in God, who created and loves me just as I am. I truly believe that I am fearfully and wonderfully made (Ps. 139:14). God has provided the means for me to lead a good life despite some disappointments. For this I am truly thankful (John 3:16).

FOR MY FRIENDS WHO SHARE POF

Kris, thirty-three, diagnosed at twenty-nine

If I could call to heaven
I would do it just for you
and ask them to watch over
and help to see you through

If I could assign an angel
to take your troubles away
I would do it without question
to brighten up your days

But I cannot call to heaven
or assign an angel to send
I can just have faith and hope for you
and always be your friend.

FOR NICHOLAS

Amy, forty-one, diagnosed at twenty-three

Years ago, in the middle of the night, I woke up and couldn't get back to sleep. Heavy on my mind was the news I had been given four years earlier: at the age of twenty-three years old I was diagnosed with premature ovarian failure. I couldn't comprehend the effect it would have on my life and the lives of the people I loved. The day of my diagnosis changed my life forever. A part of me died that day. For my husband, he knew we couldn't have any more children. My son, who was just a baby, had no idea. I would never be able to give him a brother or a sister.

That night, I got out of bed, went into the living room and sat there crying. Why did this happen? How could I cope? What would I tell my son? That is what upset me the most. My dreams included a little girl with auburn hair, whom we would name Amber Rebecca. These are my initials, too. Words kept running through my mind. So, I decided I would write my son a poem, hoping he would one day understand the most heartbreaking event of my life.

Here are the words I wrote to him on March 9, 1988:

For Nicholas

The pain I feel
is like no other
of denying you
a sister or brother

Someone to play ball with
when Mom and Dad are busy
or chase around the house
until you get dizzy

A little girl
you could call "Sis"
the pulling of pigtails
that you will miss

For God had chosen
the way it will be
as for our family
we will always be "three"

But just as the seasons
were meant to change
giving you a sibling
I cannot arrange

For if I could
I would give you a girl
someone to protect
in this great big new world

An "Amber" of light
who shines up to you
to be there in times when
life's hard to get through

Though in the midst of pain
the sun does seep through
for God gave me one chance
and that chance is—you.

I Love You, Mom

FOR YOU

Kris, thirty-three, diagnosed at twenty-nine
For my boyfriend, Dan, who was there through my POF diagnosis.

I never thought it would end this way
We both don't have a thing to say

I never felt for anyone so strong
Forever wouldn't have been too long

To start, it felt so natural and pure
I really couldn't have asked for more

I kept looking for something that wasn't there
When I should have reached out for someone to care

I didn't know how to cope at all
So I let our relationship take the fall

I obsessed over finding a key
And it finally took over the best of me

A day doesn't go by without a tear
Because losing to time is the worst to bear

I never knew what your health could cost—
But the only thing I should not have lost....

Here's to Us!

Cath, thirty-one, diagnosed at twenty-one

Although I have lived with POF for many years, I am still surprised by my own reactions to it. I was reading about other POF sufferers today, and that is what prompted me to share my story, as a cathartic way of moving forward.

My story started in 1993. I had just completed a three-year course to become a registered general nurse. It was an exciting time in my life. If I successfully completed my finals, my career would truly begin. Up to this point, life had been one huge adventure! I had many great friends in London where I trained. Those friends were who got me through this long and arduous journey.

I had felt pretty nervous prior to sitting my finals. It was a stressful time after all. I had been burning the candle at both ends, partying and studying. I was trying to find the balance to get me through the exams with a sense of humor intact, whilst performing in the exams to the best of my ability. What a sigh of relief I felt when it was over. But I had a "funny tummy" and thought I had probably given myself an ulcer with all the worry.

I went to my GP, who examined my abdomen, and this is where it all began. There, before my eyes, I saw a rounded, almost pregnant, abdomen. I explained my symptoms and my GP was quite convinced that I had become pregnant. This was news to me, since I was not seeing anyone and had not been for about eighteen months! I knew that there was no way I was pregnant and anyway, I was still having periods.

My GP proceeded to Doppler my belly in the hope of hearing a fetal heartbeat, so convinced was he that I must have lied. There was no heartbeat, as there was no pregnancy, but he decided to send me for a scan as there was a palpable mass there. I had recently lost some weight: Nothing drastic—exams are stressful! He felt it would be wise to err on the side of caution and arranged for me to have a scan. This was a scary time for me—we both knew that he felt this mass could highly likely be something suspicious. It could be cancer. I remember leaving the surgery in a daze. I felt too well, I couldn't possibly be really ill. But why was my abdomen so large? Why had my periods always been so painful that I was unable to walk, eat, or sleep for the first two days each month? I felt embarrassed. How long had my belly been this large? I didn't know. Here I was, training to become a nurse, a healthcare professional, and I couldn't even take care of my own health. I felt scared and stupid. Why hadn't I gone to the doctor sooner?

I waited a week for the scan, during which time I kept pretty busy and tried not to think too much about it. If I did I would panic! The scan showed I had one large ovarian mass. It looked like it could be a cyst, but due to my age and history, they arranged for me to have the mass removed within two weeks. The procedure was explained and I underwent the surgery. During surgery they found a second mass and severe endometriosis on my uterus, pelvis and bowel. Both cysts were successfully removed and the endometriosis lasered. I couldn't describe my utter relief on hearing the news. All was well! No cancer! Thank God!

However, five days after the surgery, things started to feel strange. I had menopausal flushing both day and night, dripping sweat, palpitations and abdominal pain. My consultant, a fantastic female surgeon who has always been open and direct with me, breezed on to the ward to examine me. She felt that the ovaries had taken a bit of battering, but should calm down in time. At this point I questioned whether the ovaries had been damaged during the procedure. She said no, they hadn't been damaged, but the surgeons had been forced to remove most of the ovarian tissue on one side as the cyst was so large. She was very reassuring and understood my concerns—the other ovary should compensate for the ovary that was not working well.

The nightmare continued for two weeks after the surgery. The pain improved, but the flushes and sweats continued and I was exhausted from sleep deprivation. I returned to my consultant and she was pretty surprised that things had not settled down. She felt the ovary was struggling and that we should rest it for a while by putting me on HRT. Instantly, my symptoms improved. The flushes were less, the sweats stopped and I felt well for the first time in many weeks—and pretty relieved.

I was kept on this medication for two months to give the ovary a good rest. When the medication was stopped, however, all of my previous symptoms returned. I was sent for scans. There was nothing abnormal detected. One ovary appeared to have been salvaged, but we came to the conclusion that it was not working. I was absolutely devastated. Prior to any of this happening, I had never been particularly interested in having a family of my own. Yes, I liked children, but other people's! I didn't really consider myself to be maternal and did not relish the idea of getting married and having a family. But when I was told that I had ovarian failure, I was devastated! I remember my consultant making some sort of hurtful quip, "If you have a sister, I would be very nice to her. You may need one of her eggs in the future." I couldn't believe it. That was it. Age twenty-one and barren. "I am afraid your ovaries do not appear to be working and we are not sure why. There is enough ovarian tissue. We cannot understand it."

And neither could I. I was distraught! I had never wanted children, but the choice had been taken away from me without discussion. This was never mentioned pre-operatively. I cannot be the only woman in the world this has happened to. They should know about the possible side effects of surgery. Why didn't they warn me? Forewarned is forearmed in my book. It wasn't fair! I was so angry! I am normally such an articulate person, calm and rarely panic, but this brought out things in me

35

that were alien. I remember leaving the hospital with my best friend, weeping and wailing. I actually scared myself. I had planned on going to the hospital on my own as it was only a checkup, but my friend had insisted she come with me. She joked that it would give me someone to chat with while I waited. Outpatient clinics never run to time. I was so grateful that she was with me. I am not sure what I would have done if she hadn't been there. My recollections of that day are very fuzzy.

I thought about the situation for many weeks. Who was I really angry with and why? The facts were that they did the surgery thinking I had cancer. I did not have cancer and there is no better news than that. The physicians acted appropriately and to the best of their abilities. It actually wasn't their fault that the ovary had packed up. I think in hindsight I was angry with myself; for being a smoker, for having severe symptoms for so long and not addressing the causes, for having an obviously larger abdomen and not going to my GP sooner. Facts are facts. At the end of the day I am alive and well. Had I been in a loving relationship I may have felt very differently about my inability to conceive. As it was I was young, free, single and intended to live life to the full.

The years passed and things carried on. My career was incredibly rewarding and life was good. Then life got even better when I met my husband in 1996. We were smitten pretty quickly and within three months I knew that I would marry this man. From the moment we met I had been open and honest about my inability to conceive, but that was never an issue. He loved me despite this. My very close friends and family knew.

Then came the story of Mrs. X who had been trying to conceive for eight million years, fifty failed IVF attempts and presto: natural conception! My friends and family tried to give me hope. It made me angry. Why couldn't they acknowledge the facts? I would never be able to conceive naturally and all the anecdotes in the world would never alter that fact. I had to deal with it, so why wouldn't they? I now understand that people were only trying to focus on being positive and probably were not sure how to deal with such an issue.

The only one who knew where I was coming from was my sister, Michelle. She had trouble conceiving and was told that she may have fertility problems. Then, suddenly, she conceived and she has the most beautiful daughter. I really couldn't love her more if she were my own. She is a joy and a delight. My sister and I have always been close, always there for each other, but sometimes that closeness can be a barrier to telling her what I really think. She is so precious to me that even now I find it very difficult to be completely honest about how I feel. She has always been very protective of me, and I think that she would feel even more guilty—she conceived and I didn't—and helpless because she cannot "fix" how I feel.

My husband and I decided we would seek advice on assisted conception. We had been trying for four years to conceive. I don't know whether you would call that denial or just optimism but you can never be totally sure of anything in life. Yes, I have ovarian failure, but what if they start to work again—it has been known to happen. After four years, we had to admit it just wasn't going to happen without some help. We sought advice, and after many tests we discovered that my husband also has fertility problems. We were told we would not conceive without ICSI, as his sperm count was low. This may sound awful, but I actually felt relived! For years I had felt a bit guilty; I would never be able to give him a family. I would never be able to pass on the good genes we have. I would always be an "unwoman" and barren.

Now I had proof that it wasn't all my fault (if fault is the word). Don't get me wrong. We were far from overjoyed about the situation, but I somehow felt that this strengthened the bond we had. I have always been fairly open and honest. "I" have fertility problems now became "we " have fertility problems. I suddenly felt less burdened. We were in this together and neither of us was to blame.

My sister did the most wonderful thing for us and donated eggs in the hope that we could conceive. That has to be the most selfless thing anyone has ever done for me. The whole affair was more traumatic than I had ever imagined and I would never undergo it again. All the counseling in the world did not prepare for me the feelings of guilt, helplessness and failure that I felt. She went through all of that for us. I had the easy part. I had the eggs implanted, but it failed. I felt pretty useless. All I had to do was act as an incubator, but my body wasn't even capable of that! She is adamant that she wants to try again, but I do not want to. I wonder if part of this is to release some of the guilt she feels at having conceived. She is far too precious for me to ever put her through anything like that again.

Today we are still hopeful that we may conceive naturally. My husband would like to give ICSI one more try, but I am not ready to even talk about that yet. We have both discussed the future without children and I feel it is in fact not as daunting as I originally thought. People find various ways of coping. Writing is my thing. I find it a cleansing way of getting my feelings out without embarrassing others. I don't think for one moment that our story is special, unusual, or particularly sad. I think it is a journey of discovery and of learning about what is important as an individual and as a wife/husband/team. I have much that is good in my life and a wonderful husband who is so caring, funny and genuine. He may not talk about things, but I know he has gone through similar feelings, and has the ability to always remain focused and positive. When I was younger, people asked me what I wanted from life. I would always say to be happy and loved, and I have that now. Children are not the be-all and end-all. I will feel cheated if I never conceive. I think we would make fantastic parents, but I won't let it rule my life and become an obsession.

OUR EGG DONATION EXPERIENCE FOLLOWING SISTER'S DIAGNOSIS OF PREMATURE OVARIAN FAILURE

Michelle, Cath's sister

I couldn't believe those years ago that Cath had had so many problems at such a young age. It then transpired that I, too, had fertility problems and was seen by the same consultant as my sister. I, too, thought the consultant was brilliant, but I always referred to my sister for a full synopsis of anyone medical since I was the nonmedical one in the family. The consultant booked me for a laparoscopy the following month and I was sent away thinking that, as advised, I would need help in fertility, but all was not lost.

The following month, my husband and I learned to our astonishment that I was pregnant, which was not in the plan for another four years, hence starting the IVF waiting list when we did. When I explained to the consultant the need to cancel my appointment for the following week she expressed both her amazement and happiness.

On May 29, 1998 at 12:05 a.m., my little girl, Hannah Catherine, was born. I couldn't believe the speedy labour and delivery, involving a trip to the toilet once at the labour ward only to discover the baby's head was dangling into the toilet, but that's another book. My husband and I are so grateful for a healthy baby.

She has brought so much happiness to us. I know that does sound like a cliché, but even though she was four years too early I was grateful that nature allowed me to give birth. Because we were so happy and grateful to have such a healthy daughter, I could not envisage my sister not being able to relish the joy herself. That is why, when hearing that discussions had taken place with the consultant regarding egg donation, we felt compelled to offer a chance for this happiness.

I was so happy to do this and didn't feel any problem with this whatsoever. The counseling sessions that followed for both my husband and me were no eye-opening experience. As far as I was concerned, Cath was my sister and she deserved more than nature was allowing. We would assist nature in any way to bring the joy of parenthood to someone so deserving.

Cath was worried about whether I had thought this through enough to warrant the time off work, traveling to and from central London from forty miles away every other day, the injections, the side effects if experienced, and if all that would be enough to extract my offer. But why would it? She is my sister. She would be a fantastic parent. She is absolutely brilliant with children and always has been (much better than myself though I am still learning).

I have suffered from rheumatoid arthritis since the birth of my daughter and discussed with the consultant halting steroid injections and reducing the medication doses I had been taking until I had completed the donation. This we both agreed to. I stopped intake of alcohol. I increased the number of visits to the gym: I needed to be in better shape for the egg donation. I needed to be both mentally and physically well, to drive through a positive attitude in the hope of rewarding the situation with success rather than dealing with the failure of all our efforts.

We proceeded with the egg donation.

I had no qualms about the injections and as it happened I was lucky enough not to experience any side effects whatsoever. This I now understand could have been due to the fact that my ovaries were not stimulated enough. I didn't mind the traveling to be reviewed for the egg growths. It was my part of the bargain and I felt pressure to achieve a good result. In order for my sister to go through all of this, I had to be able to produce good quality eggs. On the first review of the hospital scan, I was told everything looked fine. The second week I was told a few sacs filled with eggs and that they were "forming healthily." This was really exciting for both myself and Cath. I also felt under more pressure for my side of the procedure to remain in good tact if Cath was to have her chance. On my third visit, two weeks of injections later, it was decided that even though there were only half the eggs of a normal donation, they did look good, though this could only be confirmed at extraction stage and not before.

The consultant decided to go ahead and extract on the given date. I couldn't wait to get out of the ward to make the call to my sister to give her the good news.

Each time I attended the waiting room, it really hit home how this affects so many couples with so many different emotions. I would wait for my appointment and during those few minutes couples would be sitting so closely, clutching hands with white knuckles. At times I would feel sad for some of the female patients, seeing their tears rolling down their faces. Even though I had a child, it made me even more grateful that Mother Nature had allowed this, yet through no fault of these women, Nature had denied them the chance. It was also difficult to not sit there with a packet of tissues to offer to someone who was clearly emotionally torn, for fear of upsetting them more. A tissue could not console the heartache these women and couples were experiencing. That, above all, made me also realise this had to work. For Cath, it really had to work.

On the day of the extraction I was so happy to be in that ward, doing what I was doing—helping my sis become a mum. She would be a very good mother, a fantastic one, and I couldn't wait. My husband and I, and Cath and her husband met up in the waiting room. We were brought to the ward, and I was given the robe to put on, all the time joking with Cath, who seemed so nervous. In the cubicle next to me was a lady who was going through egg donation a second time. My sister and I didn't mention anything to each other about that for fear that the slightest falter on being positive would hinder the success of all our efforts.

My name was called and I walked into the theatre. I had never experienced such a friendly and relaxed atmosphere before. The nurses were smiling and so friendly. A nurse brought me to the designated bed, the lights at the viewing end were switched on and a monitor poised over the edge to report every millimetre movement of the extraction needle. Barry White was playing and I wanted the theatre to know that I was totally at ease by commenting on liking the music and opening my ankles to the sound of Barry White was indeed a first. This made the staff laugh. They even commented on how relaxed I was about the whole thing, which I had to agree with. Then, the procedure began. They explained they were in the process of inserting the needle and would be extracting any minute. I could see on the monitor what they were doing, as the needle reached further and further towards my ovaries. Excruciating pain began, and took complete control of me. This was pain I had never experienced in all my years. The pain was worse than childbirth, by far. Apparently, from this stage onwards I was put under general anaesthetic and woke up with my sister totally distraught about what had happened. To this day, I am still not sure what exactly happened. As I write this, I am a little saddened, the egg donation was not successful. There are many reasons for this, but Nature alone knows the sole reason.

I believe the clinic was at fault for many things that my sister had to go through unnecessarily, and for me going through that pain. Nobody should suffer those extremes of pain, not for childbirth and certainly not for egg donation. Now that we are wiser, we would stipulate what we would allow and what we would avoid, such as miscommunication on the results of the failure of pregnancy to my sister, and pain control at the time of extraction and after extraction for myself.

In the two years since this experience, a lot has happened in my sister's life. She is divorcing her husband and leaving the country for a one-year medical post in Australia. My first child is now four and a half years old and we are expecting our second child any day. I have had lots of ovary pain while pregnant. It's only after the donation that all the possible side effects of sensitive ovaries were discussed with various medical examiners. I have visited the local hospital where I plan to give birth, and have explained the situation in the hope of being prepared for what might be a stronger ovary pain, as well as natural pains of labour at the different stages of giving birth.

I don't mind anyone contacting me if they are thinking of doing the same as me. I am glad to be part of this by offering this small contribution so that others may try and understand what this means when contemplating such a task.

A Homework
Assignment

Susan, mother of POFer

I received a homework assignment yesterday. I haven't had homework
in years and years. My daughter, Cori, called and asked me to write a
page or two about the POF conference I attended with her a couple of
years ago. Wow, that got me thinking about so many things: not just the
conference and what it meant to me or what I learned there, but back to
1996 when Cori called us with the news that she had this condition I had
never heard of, called premature ovarian failure. Nobody I talked with
had ever heard of POF either. Well, my education was about to begin.

I think the only thing that really sunk in at that time was that she
could not have children. That was okay. Many of our friends and family members had adopted children and that is a good alternative. I
remember her talking about her doctor, the "Bimbo Babe," and how
unfeeling she was and about the medical libraries near where she lived.
I knew that any information available about POF would soon be con-
sumed by our daughter, and that knowledge shared with us. Looking
back with the wisdom that six years provides, I think I was hit with too
much information, too soon. I really thought I knew and understood
about POF, but it just couldn't all sink in.

Shortly after we moved to northern Virginia, Cori called and told us
the POF conference was going to be held near us and she and her husband would be coming for a long weekend. We were delighted! A couple

of her friends would also be staying with us. Great, the more the merrier! I would play taxi and drive them back and forth. Guess again. Cori talked me into staying for the conference and I am so thankful she did.

I found out that I didn't really have a great grasp of POF. Sure, I knew basically what it was, but listening to the doctors explain a normal cycle and what happens with POF made it all more understandable. I also learned, in a big way, that POF is much more than not being able to have children. These young women were not only experiencing symptoms of menopause, but their bodies were reacting as though they were sixty years old and these young women were scared! If their bones were becoming brittle and they were susceptible to cancer and heart conditions in their twenties and thirties, what would happen to them when they were sixty?

Emotionally, I was drained at the end of the second day. I had shed more tears, not just for Cori, but every other young woman there, than I thought possible. I listened to husbands talk about what they had been through and I listened to other mothers talk about their feelings of hopelessness in trying to help their daughters. Some said their daughters clammed up and wouldn't talk about it at all. Others said their daughters talked about it too much. We discussed the impact POF has on other family members. A session on spirituality was especially difficult; so many were questioning why, and why me.

I loved the camaraderie among these young women. I loved the way they reached out to each other and cheered every victory, large or small, whether it was improving the numbers on their bone density test, being able to exercise for an hour without hurting, or learning about an adoption about to take place. I loved how they shared e-mail addresses to help support each other after the conference and encouraged each other to come back next year and bring someone. I loved how they wanted to reach out to those who weren't there and those who didn't know about the conference. I loved how they wanted to educate their own medical personnel.

In my heart, I'm very sorry the conference will not be here this year.

Not only will we not get that extra week-end with our daughter, but I won't be seeing the young women whom I admire so much. In my head, I'm delighted for those young women who will have the opportunity to participate in the conference this year.

HOPE

Josette, thirty-three, diagnosed at twenty-eight

The first time I heard the words premature ovarian failure, I thought nothing of it. A reproductive endocrinologist was throwing jargon at me as I was getting dressed after a hysterosalpingography.

My father had taken me to the doctor's office that day and was driving me to my regular gynecologist appointment, which immediately followed. I mentioned this to my father and we both shrugged. The doctor never bothered to explain to me what the ramifications of this diagnosis were.

During my gynecological appointment, I casually mentioned this to my doctor. He looked at me long and hard with a very concerned look on his face and asked, "Do you know what that means? That means you would never be able to have a baby on your own. The only options open to you would be adoption or a donor egg."

As everything went white, I saw my dreams shattering. How could this be? What did I do to deserve this curse? I will not accept this. Why didn't my doctor see this coming? Why is life so unfair? They have to be wrong…I'm only twenty-eight years old…Why don't you just tell me I have cancer? Please stop this noise…

Needless to say, I was not handling this news very well, and once it was confirmed, I was truly on the verge of a nervous breakdown. My husband would come home from work nightly to find me crying hysterically. My parents would come over every day to keep me occupied, preventing my mind from wandering back to this terrible reality I could

49

not escape. I thought about traveling to Medjugorje where I heard people get miraculously cured. I saw doctor after doctor who told me the same thing. I spoke to a priest and called prayer lines.

Even my husband, my rock, the person from whom I drew my strength to deal with this terrible "mistake," lost his hold on his emotions one night as we lay in bed. Never before did I think how horrible this was for him as well. Did he deserve to lose out on a family because my body was, as I saw it, prematurely "rotting?" I always knew getting pregnant would not be an easy feat, as my periods were irregular and unpredictable. I even told him when we talked about getting married that we might have problems. But this?

To add insult to injury, many of my friends and co-workers were expecting. The mere hint of someone being pregnant sent me into crying fits that would last the entire day. I could not focus on work and I began to suffer socially, as I could not bear to see my friends' bellies begin to swell. Going to baby showers was out of the question.

We were also beginning to feel the financial burden of fertility treatment. How were we going to handle the costs of Pergonal and Lupron? The insurance would cover up to $10,000 for IVF (if I ever got to that point), but that amount would be exhausted very quickly.

A friend of my mother worked for a fertility doctor and she begged me to try him. My husband and I went only to meet a pompous jerk who used me as a teaching lesson for a student doctor who was observing. Without even giving me an examination or drawing blood he began to draw diagrams to explain how we are born with a certain amount of eggs and we begin to lose them as early as when we are in utero. I had "none left."

We left his office feeling defeated once again and after a good long cry I decided that I wanted a baby and would be open to the possibility of a donor egg. I discussed this option with my sisters and they both gladly offered to help. I felt a great weight lifted off of my chest. This was the hand that was dealt me, but it did not mean I could not pursue my dreams of a family.

I began to feel more positive about the future and I started to have more fun. I went to parties and weddings and even went out for drinks with my husband and friends. Instead of approaching intimacy as if it were a job, my husband and I began to enjoy ourselves again. I felt something changing in me, but could not put my finger on it. I was going to one more doctor to confirm that my only means of having children would be through a donor egg.

He was a highly recommended doctor and I felt greatly relieved that our efforts were not in vain when he told me he was not completely convinced that I could not conceive on my own. He ran the usual work-up and advised me I would hear from him within a week.

In a week's time, he called advising me that I ovulated and I should expect a period within the next week or two. You can imagine how happy I was. The others were wrong. Within a week I started to feel like I was coming down with the flu. I had constant headaches, body aches and I was very tired. Taking pregnancy tests once a month was no novelty to me since I didn't get a period. I guess it was wishful thinking. This time, however, it was more than that: it was a reality. I took a test on Valentine's Day morning and it showed positive. I thought there was something wrong with it and my husband suggested I take a second test. The sheer joy that I felt was unbelievable. First, I called my entire family (they all thought I was having a false pregnancy and questioned my sanity), then I left an emergency message for the doctor. He sent me for blood work and when he called me to confirm that I was pregnant I heard disbelief in his voice. "According to your records this can't happen. This is a miracle. You should write a book." My prayers were answered and I would finally know happiness.

I gave birth to a healthy girl and I thought, "Those doctors didn't know what they were talking about. Now my body will go back to normal and I'm going to have five kids."

I soon learned that I was wrong and the doctors were right when I went right back to missing periods after the birth of my daughter. My regular gynecologist once again told me I would not be able to conceive again because I had no eggs left. I knew I had to go to alternative sources for more information on this condition and turned to the Internet. I was delightfully shocked when I found a site that was a support group for women with the same problem I had. I had always thought I was alone with this horrible secret. Through this site, I learned more about my condition and I believe I understand it more than my doctor does.

Still, I longed for another child and so I turned to alternative medicine and saw an acupuncturist to try to stimulate my ovaries. I did not take medicine, but I did take Chinese herbs and after four months found out I was pregnant again. I unfortunately could not hold this pregnancy and miscarried within a week of finding out. The loss of this pregnancy was devastating to me, but it could not compare to the suffering I went through when I was first diagnosed with premature ovarian failure. That seemed like a death sentence. This was a very sad time in my life, but I know how fortunate and blessed I am to have had a child.

Today, I'm thirty-three years old and while I am still trying to get pregnant again, I now know it is more important to keep my body healthy. I know I need estrogen and progesterone replacement to keep my bones and heart healthy and to increase the probability of conceiving. I also know I can go in and out of premature ovarian failure and that I do have a chance at getting pregnant again over the next few years. I have my faith and love from family and friends. I know there are worse fates than this and I know I am not alone.

A Husband's Story

David. This first appeared in the POFSG newsletter,

Endless POFibilities—December 2000

in the column, POF Point of View: A Husband's Story

My name is David. I'm Cori Canty's husband. Cori and I were married in May of 1995. Before we married she knew there might be some problem with reproducing, since she'd had only two periods since age fourteen. I don't remember if she told me before or after we got married. I do remember that I didn't see it as a major obstacle. My focus of marriage has been Cori and myself, and our relationship. The hardest thing to deal with has been trying to help Cori come to terms with her POF. It has been tough to comfort her when she feels incomplete and defective (her words, not mine). As a male and a husband, I don't see her as either. I see her as human. We all have problems and difficulties to deal with and overcome. As a husband, my role is to support her as she struggles through difficulties. Her role is to do the same for me.

I do have a different perspective on starting a family. I would like to have a family of my own. As far as what "my own" means, I can only offer my viewpoint. My own family will be Cori, myself, and any kids that we raise, take care of, and support. These kids can be from donor egg, adoption, or any other method of having children, whatever that may be.

I know other males and females may feel different. They want to have their own kids from their own reproductive systems... I hope I'm being clear. This is a conflict people must deal with on their own. I realize Cori and I cannot have children the way many other people do, so we have to find other ways. I have accepted this. Cori seems to be resigned to this fact after hearing her latest results. It took her many years before being able to "accept" this. Hopefully, I have been supportive of her in the struggle. All I can say is I've tried my best.

Cori also mentioned that some women were worried about being single and having POF or infertility problems. I'm not sure I can offer much help since I can only offer my perspective. I wasn't looking for the perfect person to marry. If I had found the perfect person, I would have to be perfect, which I'm not. I was looking for someone with whom I was compatible. I expected Cori to be human and have problems and difficulties to overcome. I knew that I was and did…still do. Anyway, from this point of view, having POF or other infertility problems is just another difficulty to overcome. This goes back to when Cori told me about her problem. I didn't look at it as a defect or something that made her less of a woman, just human.

I feel lucky that I have been able to support Cori in her struggle to come to terms with her POF. I know it would be tough for her to go through it alone (although she would have the support of her online friends).

I'm in What!!

Stacey, forty, diagnosed at thirty-four

"You have to hurry," was my gynecologist's response to my question: "Can I have children?" He had just told me that my blood tests indicated my hormones were elevated. I recall he mentioned certain words and letters—which, at the time, I did not understand—indicating the onset of menopause had arrived. It was January 28, 1998, two days before my thirty-fifth birthday, and I had just been told I was in "perimenopause."

I thought, "How can this be? This can't be happening! I just got married five months ago and I'm not quite thirty-five years old!"

Now, I realize these thoughts were not unlike those of many other women who undergo premature ovarian failure before they've been able to start a family, but at the time I felt like the most alone person in the world. There were several reasons for this: both of my parents were recently deceased, this conversation with my doctor took place over the telephone, at a time when I was home alone, and I had never heard of anyone being menopausal before turning thirty-five!

By the time I was diagnosed with POF, I felt that life had dumped a lot of unhappy circumstances upon me.

That is not to say that nothing had gone right in the recent past. I had met a guy whom I really loved and who really loved me, too. He stood by me while I grieved the loss of my mother and while I cared for my dying father. A little more than a year after we met, we married (and I walked myself down the aisle). We started trying to have a family right

55

away, and at my annual visit with my gynecologist, he discovered a large cyst by my left ovary. Three months after I was married, I had surgery for endometriosis and lost a piece of my left ovary. That was okay; I still had my right ovary, and I could feel it functioning every month, or at least I used to be able to feel it function. At that time, I remember telling my doctor that I felt I had not ovulated in several months. I was assured nothing was wrong and accepted the advice without further question.

Two months later, in January 1998, I began getting severe hot flashes and couldn't ignore the symptoms any longer. I had started getting occasional hot flashes in January 1997 and missing periods once in a while, but I thought, "Who wouldn't after all I had been through?" I chalked it all up to stress and didn't give it another thought…until the hot flashes really picked up. I realized I had not felt "right" for quite some time and got scared. I could hardly believe my ears when my gynecologist said yes, it was possible I was entering menopause. As I said earlier, when the diagnosis was confirmed, I felt my (new) world falling apart.

My gynecologist referred me to two reproductive endocrinologists who maintained donor egg programs. He told me that would be the route I'd likely have to take to bear children. I remember thinking it just could not be possible that I was the end of my parent's joint gene pool. I was the only child they'd had together although each had children from previous marriages. It also seemed incredibly cruel that I could not pass down parts of my parents forever in my own children. In addition to grieving my parents' loss, I also had to grieve the loss of my own children. I spent two full days in bed before summoning the strength to go back to work and start living again.

Once I started to get back on my feet, I did what I typically do when I don't know what is going on…I educate myself. I went to the library and looked for books on menopause. What I found was extremely disappointing. There were no books for people like me. In fact, there weren't even chapters in books for people like me. All of the information discussed menopause as an event that occurs as women near fifty, and none treated it as the terrible turn of events I viewed it as. I remember one author saying women in their fifties may be able to laugh about the symptoms with their mother who went through "the change" decades before. This was particularly upsetting because I was in my mid-thirties and I didn't have a mother to talk this over with.

Even more upsetting was what I began learning about estrogen and how deleterious its loss is for women, particularly as we live longer and longer without it. I thought, "my God, my body is going through this change at least ten years earlier that it should and it's bad for me to boot!" My body seemed so delicate and so old.

At the same time, I began working with two fertility facilities, one from which I was receiving fertility drugs while waiting to move up the list for an egg donor and one with which I was just waiting for an egg donor. As it turned out, my ovaries did not stimulate very well and the attempts at insemination failed. Although having my hopes go up and down each month was very difficult, I don't think I was ready to admit to myself that maybe I really would not be able to have a baby with my genes. That started to change as the summer wore on, and at some point I realized that if I really wanted to have a baby, I'd have to give up on the dream of looking for my father's hair and my mother's eyes in my child. My husband was supportive throughout everything.

It was just about that time that we became lucky on the donor front and received the profile of a donor whom we liked. By the time we agreed to accept the donor, I knew I was doing the right thing, and I never had a single question in my mind from that point forward. We proceeded with the program, and on September 11, 1998 my son was conceived. He was transferred into my womb on September 14 and was born on May 31, 1999. My son is unquestionably the most important and wonderful thing that has ever happened in my life. It is impossible to put into words the love I feel for him and awe he invokes in me every single day. My husband and I are truly blessed.

It's been more than three years since I was diagnosed with POF, and I'm very happy to say that a lot has changed. For one thing, there are at least two books and two Websites devoted to the issue. These are truly gifts of immense proportions as they may help other women avoid some of the intense loneliness I experienced. Additionally, menopause now is a topic covered routinely on the news, on talk shows and even in advertisements. There is even an occasional mention of women undergoing menopause early. The information available about HRT has grown by leaps and bounds. These are all positive developments.

I am still struggling with the death of my parents, and once again am trying to come to grips with the death of my fertility. On February 13 of this year, I was diagnosed with an ectopic pregnancy, which was terminated surgically about five hours later. This felt like someone had played the cruelest joke in the world on me. Miraculously, I was pregnant, but I could not carry that baby to term. That episode sent me spiraling down an emotional roller coaster that lasted for several weeks. Intense therapy, with a social worker who has seen me through all of my difficult times since 1994, helped me deal with this loss as well.

But it now seems that our luck is turning around again. Two weeks ago, our long wait for another egg donor came to an end, and we are about to embark upon that journey once again. Will we be fortunate enough to be blessed with another wonderful child? We certainly hope so. But even if we're not, we know that we are still incredibly lucky to have our son.

I'M NOT ALONE

Shelly, forty-eight, diagnosed at thirty-eight

I have had female health problems since the age of seventeen. First, there were irregular periods and then, ovarian cysts. I was in extreme pain the summer before my senior year of high school. I remember my mother asking me if I wanted to go to church camp or to the hospital for tests. I opted for the hospital. She was concerned listening to me cry myself to sleep every night. During surgery the doctor removed a cyst the size of a large orange on my right ovary, another one half the size on my left ovary, my appendix which was upside down and a diverticulum on my small intestine.

I then had three miscarriages in three years. I was devastated with the first one. What had I done to cause this? After the third miscarriage I underwent a barrage of tests. The results indicated I was borderline low on progesterone.

Later, I would experience endometriosis. I had laproscopic surgery three times to remove the endometriosis. During the last surgery my doctor removed my right ovary because it had hemorrhaged and was adhered upside down to the backside of my uterus. I really wanted to have children, but my hopes were diminishing.

My periods became irregular and every time I called the doctor she ordered a pregnancy test to make sure I wasn't pregnant—I knew most of the pregnancy tests would be negative—then she would prescribe medication to start my periods. I had also started experiencing a low libido. Next came the hot flashes. I asked my husband the infamous question, "Is it hot in here or is it me?" His reply would always be, "It's you, honey." Oh, and let's not talk about the weight gain!

My doctor decided it would be a good idea to check my FSH level about every four months. When I went in for my yearly exam she gave me the news: premature ovarian failure. What? I'm too young for this. We briefly discussed egg donation and she gave me the name of a doctor. At the same time we found out that we would be moving temporarily, so the egg donation was put on hold.

When my doctor gave me the news that I would have a really slim chance of conceiving I was devastated. I called my husband at work crying and he said not to worry, we can adopt, but I wanted to have our own children! For the next couple of years we talked about adoption, but never pursued it.

I have tried several different types of hormone replacement therapy. I am currently taking a break from it. I feel as though I have been cheated out of having my own children. I try to tell myself that God must have other plans for me. I still feel as though I have missed out on a beautiful experience. To tell you the truth, some days I feel like a freak. All of my friends have children. What is wrong with me? So, imagine my excitement and relief to know there is a whole group of us POFers! Once again, I'm not alone.

IT'S IN BIGGER HANDS
THAN MINE

Lori, thirty-four, (re)diagnosed at thirty-two

My story started at age eighteen. That's when I had the last natural period of my life. It was my freshman year at college, September 1987. I had no idea why I didn't get my period in October, November, or December. I started gaining weight, but attributed it to the "Freshman 15." I went on a diet in January and lost all the weight I had gained; but still no period. In April, I finally went to the campus medical center for my first gynecological exam only to be told it was stress and not to worry about it. My libido went to zero; I was irritable and moody; I was constantly having "hot flashes." I now realize, at age thirty-two, that I was going through menopause at eighteen. I finally told my parents and went to my doctor at home during summer break. He put me on BCP for a month as a test to see if they would induce a period and they worked. I was immediately referred to a gynecologist and an endocrinologist who put me through numerous blood/thyroid tests. The end result that was explained to me was that I had "auto immune ovarian failure" and my ovaries weren't functioning. I was then told that perhaps I would have difficulty having children, "but don't worry about it now, just keep taking BCPs and you will be fine."

So, throughout the rest of my college years and my twenties, I never thought about it again...until I was thirty-one and my husband and I started talking about having our own children. I stopped taking BCPs, and my period stopped as well. My gynecologist immediately put me on HRT and referred me to an RE. On Sept. 13, 2001, I was officially (re)diagnosed with premature ovarian failure. It was a harsh reality to face this diagnosis at thirty-two, when having a child was our next step. Our only options were donor egg or adoption. Since I have two sisters who volunteered to be donors, we decided to pursue the DE route first. My first DE cycle was in February 2002; everything went well up until the retrieval. My sister had an adverse reaction to the anesthesia and was in severe pain postsurgery. It was heart-wrenching for me to see her in such pain. Three days later I had my transfer and twelve days after that, I went in for my beta-hCG test. On March 7, 2002, I had my first set of bad news; it was negative. My husband and I decided to take a few months off and travel. Immediately upon our return from Italy, we decided to do our FET with the remaining embryos. On June 28, 2002 we had the transfer. On July 10, it was negative again. We were very disappointed and emotionally drained by the entire process. We are taking a year off before we start all over again with my youngest sister. In the meantime, we are starting to pursue international adoption. Time will tell what the outcome will be. It's in bigger hands than mine.

LEARNING TO TRUST

Elizabeth, forty-four, diagnosed at sixteen

I was diagnosed with POF when I was sixteen years old. I was not reaching puberty like my peers. My mother took me to the doctor, who then referred me to an endocrinologist. This was back in 1975 when there was no Internet and no proliferation of the support groups we have today.

After strange and intrusive tests, the doctor delivered the bad news. I numbed out and felt very strange and disconnected. The doctor simply told me to not cry anymore, tell no one. You cannot have children. Take these pills and you will develop like the other girls. One insensitive male resident even told me, when asked if the pills would work, "These pills would make even me grow breasts." How's that for bedside manner? A social worker was dispatched, trying to help me, but my mother waved her off, "She's too upset to talk."

Funny, no one asked me. No one asked me anything. Looking back, I believe my mother could not deal with the diagnosis and did what my family traditionally did with anything unpleasant; buried it under the rug. A lot of the family's pain was buried under this rug.

My family acted as if nothing happened. A wall of shame and silence was erected. That night my family went shopping for a family car. I felt saddled with shame and was unable to discuss it with them. Even as an adult when I tried to talk to my mother she would say, "How do you think I feel?" I asked her if my father knew and she sadly said yes. I asked her what he said, and she said he cried.

In college I never tried to date or find my soulmate because, as I reasoned, life had dealt me out of that game. I became involved with the party scene, blocking out life with drugs, alcohol, and unfulfilling relationships. I dated a lot of men, but I pledged never, ever, to get close to anyone. I told everyone that I did not want to get married. I lied. I told everyone that I did not want to have children. I lied again, and lived this lie for many years. Discontentment, unfulfilled dreams and depression were a way of life. Worse, I lost any faith in the God I had learned about as child. As I figured it, God must have known I would be a terrible mother and spared some poor child from being born. When women got married or had children a dull ache resonated inside. I was never taught how to accept this diagnosis—this sentence—or even to accept it as reality. I didn't deal with it. I never allowed myself to feel the pain.

I fell in love for the first time when I was forty with a man who had been married and had a child. I pushed him away as was my usual custom, but his gentleness and loving spirit drew me to him. I took a chance and let myself fall in love. When I told him about my "biological sentence" he was very supportive and accepting. At times I wanted him to find someone else, anyone else, because I did not feel like a whole woman, but he remained at my side and helped me to begin to heal.

When I was forty-one my mother's doctor thought she had cancer. Being the loving and dutiful daughter, I explored the Internet for answers. I found the best doctors in the United States and pledged my help for her. I was determined to overturn her sentence! I told her to spend any inheritance she was to pass on to her children on her treatment. I wanted my mother to be alive and well. We learned later she did not have cancer, but she had a situation that warranted "watchful waiting." This search for help for my mother and the love of the man in my life brought me to the next step in the healing process.

After my mother's cancer scare, somewhere deep inside a voice spoke to me. The God whom I loved as a child, yet I believed had abandoned me in my time of despair, said to me, "What about you? What about your premature ovarian failure diagnosis? Are there any answers? Or is it really like the doctors told you, there is no hope?" I decided to check out the Internet again, this time on my behalf. I entered "premature ovarian failure" into a search engine and found the POF support group. To be quite honest, I was shocked that it even existed, since the doctors made it sound so freakish. I remember I started to cry. I was finally crying the tears I was told to never cry. Other women suffered from this disease as well! I learned that this disease can affect other parts of my body and became very angry at the medical establishment and my family for their negligence. Finally, as I found myself already in this healing state of consciousness, this newly found anger propelled me into positive action. This was the first healthy thing I did about my POF in my entire life.

I attended a local support group, and after four meetings finally accepted my diagnosis, reached out for support, became empowered, and even plan on going to the NIH for some answers. This is progress, progress for the girl who would hide and deny her diagnosis. I've met other women just like me and for the first time in my life do not feel alone. I am now cohosting a chat for teens who are diagnosed with POF. I want to help teens and their parents get through this and get the information they need so they can lead full lives. POF owned me before. Now I not only want not to own it, but help others to gain ownership. I met a woman from another state who, like myself, was diagnosed as a teen and also came from a family that was not supportive. We share so many of the same feelings of alienation. It is truly healing to be there for one another. We keep in touch and offer support on many of life's issues.

This support group has changed my life and has begun to give me some hope; something that was extinguished when I received my diagnosis in 1975. Most importantly, I know POF is not a life sentence. I will never know what my life could have been had I received the support I needed as a teen, but I have to believe that as long as I walk through this pain and use all of the resources that the POF support group offers I will be happier. Once again, as when I was child, I dare to dream again. I now know and admit I want to be a mother. I was denied the chance to pass on my genetic material, but I can adopt and be a mother.

LIVING WITH POF

Marrianne, forty-three, diagnosed at sixteen

I was diagnosed with primary ovarian failure at age sixteen. I have lived with this diagnosis and have been on hormone replacement therapy for twenty-five years. I hope that my story might help others who have been diagnosed with this rare form of premature ovarian failure.

I grew up as many girls did, looking forward to the time when I would be a mother to my own children. I would pretend to be pregnant with a pillow or dolly under my shirt. I also grew up in an atmosphere where marrying, being a mother, and raising children was a large part of who I would be. This was reinforced by my religious community. My parents raised me as early as age six with information about where babies came from and how they developed in a woman. As I grew older I learned about my body maturation. In seventh grade, I looked forward to the day I would have my first period along with my friends.

Over time there became a marked difference between my peers and me in our physical sexual development. I had a "fat pad" on my stomach region and because my breasts were so undeveloped, I was teased and taunted by others. They claimed I was pregnant; ironically an experience I would never have. I was very naïve and very virginal.

Late in my fourteenth year my wise mother became concerned about my lack of maturation and delayed menstruation, and took me to my pediatrician. The doctor discounted my mother's concerns, saying I was just "a late bloomer," but my mother couldn't understand how I began enough breast development to wear a training bra and then at age

67

twelve everything stopped. I did not have any signs of appropriate body hair or spotting. Mom decided to get a second opinion. After one thorough exam by another well-recommended doctor, I was immediately sent to the pediatric endocrine clinic at Johns Hopkins Hospital in Baltimore, Maryland, not far from our home. I will forever be grateful for my mother's persistence.

After many examinations and tests, it was determined that I needed hormone replacement therapy. My parents worried over this decision, but I'm happy to say they chose to start. They worried about the effect the medication would have on me, especially taking it at such a young age. My FSH levels were over 1,000 and I had infantile development. My bone age had a two-year lag, even though my chromosomes tested normal. I didn't realize it at the time but being on hormone replacement therapy was vital to my physical womanly development and a part of my sexual happiness in marriage. The doctors started me out on very low doses and gradually increased the amount, monitoring my development. I have now been on them nearly twenty-five years.

My sister, five years younger than I, started developing early and had her first period before me. She was less prepared for it, because I was no example to her. I had mixed emotions about her being first. I was a bit jealous, but I also had a tremendous sense of relief, feeling that she would be normal and wouldn't need to endure what I was experiencing.

In my sixteenth year I was treated at the gynecology clinic at Johns Hopkins. It was then that I heard of my diagnosis. The doctor indicated to my mother in my presence that I had an extremely rare condition called primary amenorrhea, also known as primary ovarian failure with unknown origin. As he explained my diagnosis to her, a wave of shock hit me. I understood enough to realize that something was seriously wrong. I piped us and asked, "Are you saying that I won't be able to have children?"

He told me it was unlikely, and that if I wanted to have children I would have to adopt them. He said that my body most likely did not have sufficient eggs in my ovaries or at least didn't have enough "good" ones, to conceive. They could not find a reason for this failure. Since a woman is born with all the eggs she will ever have, the doctor said conception was highly unlikely in my case. However, they couldn't be certain unless I had an ovarian biopsy. The doctors were split about whether I should be biopsied or not. My parents were more concerned about how this blow would affect me psychologically than about my reproductive future, so I was never biopsied. After hearing about my diagnosis, tears welled up in my eyes, and anything else the doctor may have said after that eluded me.

After my appointment, I spent the next thirty minutes riding home in the car playing the doctor's words over and over in my mind. I was already not like other girls and now I was being told that I would not be like other women either. Was this for real? When I got home I asked Mom to tell me again what the doctor had said. I needed to hear it from her lips, too. Then I went into my bedroom and cried.

As I began sharing my POF diagnosis with a few close friends, they had a difficult time understanding how my just being female wouldn't make it possible. "You'll have children," they would say in consolation, and then they would just let it go as if my problem had been solved. I felt very alone with my diagnosis. I knew someone who had adopted a baby after trying for seven years and then got pregnant. This is what my friends expected for me.

When I started dating, I kept quiet about my POF until we became serious about possible marriage. Some of my boyfriends just passed it off, as if it was no big deal, but the man I finally married took it seriously. He responded in a caring, nurturing way, and shed a few tears with me. At one point we did split up, but not over this. While we were apart, he learned to love another woman's child, but fortunately not the other woman. He returned to me knowing he could love a child other than his own flesh and blood.

He was in the military and, after marrying, we were stationed in

Guam. One time while there, all the wives on our street and the street behind us were pregnant at the same time. It was a standing joke that it was " in the water," and I wasn't drinking enough. I was having a hard enough time dealing with all the new birth announcements from friends back home, but this was too much. To make matters worse, I missed my husband terribly while he was deployed and was truly alone dealing with this. I came to a breaking point when my close friend on my street had her baby. I wanted to be happy for her, but I was too jealous. When I held the baby, I had sweet feelings, but when I went home empty handed to an empty, childless home, it was more than I could bear. I fell to my knees and prayed to God for comfort and help in dealing with this cross I had to bear. Feelings of comfort poured over me as I prayed and cried.

After two years of marriage, I inquired about adoption through our church's social service program. We would be returning to the states and would be perfect candidates for adoption. Three months later, my husband was in a military air accident that took his life and our opportunity to have a family.

After being widowed for four years, I met and married my current husband. He already had two teenage boys. To stave off possible resentment, I agreed before we married that I would not "parent" them. I kept my word, but it was hard for me to figure out just how to fit in the family. I wanted to be more than just friends. Over time I have grown to feel like family, and my stepsons have accepted me as such, for which I am grateful. I wanted to be a mom and feel more like a mom, so my husband and I pursued adoption for over ten years without success. When grandchildren came along, I wondered again how I would fit in. We were fortunate enough to live close by, allowing me to bond with them.

After the second grandchild came, my daughter-in-law asked me if I felt like the children's grandmother. She hoped that I did, because I had given a grandmother's love to them. For a long time I felt love as family, but I felt more like a close aunt. I was able to make a greater transition to Grandma because I had been acknowledged as such. That acknowledgment meant so very much to me. Being a grandmother at forty is helping me make the transition of not having children of my own. I have been able to care for my grandchildren in many aspects, from infancy on up. I am grateful that I did not allow the roller coaster ride of adoption or POF to get in the way of loving the family I am blessed to be a part of. Though I have not experienced every aspect, I have been able to share and grow in the roles I play in my family members' lives. I have had more regular, ordinary days living with POF than not. I have found it important to accept whatever grief or pain comes up. I usually journal my feelings or talk about them with a close friend. For various reasons, hi-tech considerations, such as *in vitro* fertilization, were not options for us. The doctor's easy answer of adoption, which we pursued, was not so easy for us. After trying numerous approaches for over ten years, we felt it was time to stop. Many doors closed to us for various reasons not in our control. It is critical to start these procedures as early as possible. I know many have had wonderful experiences, but as with everything, there are no guarantees.

Not working on having a child is still new to me. I still get twinges of disappointment and discomfort when I see other pregnant women, or when I see mothers holding their infants. I have felt less lonely in my situation as I have visited the POF support board on the Internet. I appreciate the opportunity of connection, learning, and helping others more like myself.

I am learning to add a little bit more of what I love doing, still giving and sharing with others to fill my life. I have many questions to ask God when I leave this world. Until then, I choose to keep going and doing the best I can.

Michael and Zach

(my nephews, ages two and one)

Kris, thirty-three, diagnosed at twenty-nine

The most precious things I'll ever know
I thank God that I will see them grow

In blood they'll be the closest thing to me
I struggle to let go of what else could be

I wasn't blessed to have my own
So I'll learn to be satisfied with just a loan

It hurts sometimes to see them smile
I pray this will pass after a while

I try to think this is part of a plan
And strive to rise above as best I can

I try to imagine the love they feel
And I hope I will feel it just as real

I hope they know how lucky they are
Because for me this gift is so very far

My Experience with Premature Ovarian Failure

Lisa, thirty-four, diagnosed at twenty-nine

My name is Lisa and I am now thirty-two years old. My troubles began when I was beginning the puberty transition. I would get my period one month and then not again for three months. I could never count on my period coming when I thought it should.

My mother took me to the doctor when I was sixteen. He took blood to do hormone tests and said everything was fine. This went on for a while, then I went to a doctor who said that this was not normal, so he put me on birth control pills to regulate me. They regulated me for as long as I took them, but when I went off of them, my period stopped again. I took them for three months, went off of them, and did not get my period for three months. My doctor put me on Provera to jump-start my body. I took Provera for five days and then I got my period. I have repeatedly tried birth control pills and Provera, but they never did the trick. I have gone through Pap tests since I was sixteen. My doctor always said my uterus was very small. All of the Pap tests I have ever had were normal.

When I was twenty-four I started taking birth control pills again, this time for a year. I then went off of them and for the six months I was studying in Germany I did not get a period.

I was in Austria (now twenty-six) studying for my master's degree, and I was feeling tired all of the time. I found a lump in my neck and went to three doctors there and they all thought it was nothing.

I returned to the United States after the summer of 1995. I went to three more doctors here and not one would test me for anything. I felt something was wrong, so I went to my small-town doctor. He checked my neck and said it was my thyroid. He ran some tests, including a needle biopsy, and I was diagnosed with papillary cancer of the thyroid. I went through tests, surgery, and radiation treatment.

Since I had come back to the United States, my periods had stopped. They were fine while I was in Austria. We thought it might just be from the stress and trauma.

After the surgery, my parathyroids did not function, so my calcium level dropped. I could have died from that since calcium controls the muscles. My parathyroids do not currently work, so I am on a high dose of calcium and Rocaltrol.

I was treated for the cancer from October through December of 1995. No periods. I went back to my doctor. He took some blood to do hormone tests. He came back in the room, and said, "Your FSH is really high, in postmenopausal range."

I said, "What does that mean?"

He asked me if I was planning on having kids. I said not at the time, and he proceeded to tell me I would never have kids. I felt bad at the time, not feeling like a real woman. Real women are supposed to be able to have babies.

Two years passed. Two years with no periods. Not that I am really complaining. I did not have cramps or the need for supplies. I was twenty-nine. I decided that it was time to really find out what was happening. I went to an endocrinologist in Milwaukee. He tested my hormone levels again. Again the FSH was in postmenopausal range. He told me I would not be able to have kids. We tried to find out why this had happened by testing the immune system for autoimmune diseases. Along with the thyroid cancer, I had the early stages of Hashimoto's

Thyroiditis, which is an autoimmune disease. My immune system seemed fine. He said he had not had a lot of these cases and that most of the time, you never find out what the problem is. Nothing was showing us the cause.

Later, he went to a convention and while there, he brought up my case to other doctors. They talked about different possibilities like genetic disorders such as Turner syndrome and other diseases that could cause this. He told me I did not have Turner's because I did not look like a person with Turner's, but he did a karyotype just to rule it out. They took blood, and did the karyotype. I got a call from him saying that I was missing one half of one of my X chromosomes and that it turns out I have Turner syndrome. This happens when all or part of an X chromosome is missing. Only one in twenty-five hundred female births have this.

They got me in to see a geneticist right away for counseling. She went over with me what the signs are, and why it happened. She talked to me about the symptoms of Turner's and what could happen with the missing part of the chromosome. Soft nails, weak eye muscles, cancer, and premature ovarian failure were listed. It is not genetic. My parents did not give this to me. For some reason, the X chromosome gets lost in the cells as they divide. I found out that Turner's can cause some types of cancer, can alter eyesight, and can cause diabetes. Since I am not full-blown, I may or may not get some of the stuff associated with Turner's. I believe the thyroid cancer was a part of it. The cancer led me to find this out.

My endocrinologist referred me to a good gynecologist who made me feel comfortable right away. I had a regular yearly exam and as I was making almost no estrogen on my own, she started me on HRT. She prescribed the estrogen in the form of a patch. I used them, but the dose was too high. I was crying all the time. I called her and told her about the depression and uncontrolled crying. She lowered the dosage of the patch, but it was still too high. She ended up giving me Prempro, the lowest dose of progesterone she could find.

I have been on Prempro for a few years now. I have no major side effects and I don't even get my period. Again, I am really not complaining! Now I just go in to see her for my yearly exam.

My endocrinologist scans me for thyroid cancer every year. I have been clean for six years. He also works to keep my calcium level up. I am at high risk of osteoporosis. All of these things come full circle. I don't make estrogen, and I don't make calcium—I could lose so much bone density. Because I don't make calcium, I take high doses of calcium citrate, so hopefully I will be okay in the years to come. Also, I had a bone density test and it came back fine.

Going through all of this was devastating. I was angry about the cancer thing and that the doctors would not listen to me. After I found out I could not have kids, I thought I was not really a woman. After I found out about the Turner syndrome I thought I was a freak of nature. For a long time, I denied I had any problems.

In the past year, I have started looking at my life. I have two cats that serve as my kids. I have two nephews and one niece who serve as my kids. My mother instinct is taken care of. I feel I am too old to adopt. I always wanted to have kids young so I would have more in common with them. I started volunteering with the Person to Person Network for the Thyroid Cancer Survivor's Association. I have found that talking about my issues helps me deal with them. The Turner's thing I am still working on. Sometimes I wonder, am I a guy? Well, I know I am not. I am a lucky person who is still here to tell her story.

Sometimes people look at me as if I am making this up. So many serious things can't happen to one person. Well, I tell you they can and they did to me. I am a much better person having gone through what I have, and I am much stronger. I know now that I don't have to believe that a doctor is God. I know my body better than anyone else. If they don't believe me, I will just find someone who does.

Thank you for listening to my story. I want to make sure that I tell everyone one more thing. Be sure to touch yourself. I know it sounds bad, but touch yourself. Know what your body feels like. If I had not been touching my neck I would not have found the lump and may not be here today.

I told my general practitioner that I needed a medical bracelet to warn others about my medical problems. He said, "You don't need a bracelet, you need an attaché case!"

MY GALACTOSEMIA STORY

Stacey, twenty-six

I was born February 16, 1977 in London, Ontario, Canada. I was the first baby born in ten years at the hospital with a rare genetic disease known as galactosemia. At this time there was little information on galactosemia. There were also no newborn screenings. Galactosemia is an inherited disease in which the transformation of galactose to glucose is blocked, causing galactose to increase to toxic levels in the body. High levels of galactose can cause vomiting, diarrhea, lethargy, low blood sugar, brain damage, jaundice, liver enlargement, cataracts, susceptibility to infection and even death. In adults with galactosemia, symptoms include speech disorders, cataracts, ovarian atrophy and infertility, and behavioral problems.

In my case, I was diagnosed at six weeks of age while clinging to life. My liver was literally the size of a football. I had jaundice, bleeding through the skin, and one dense cataract due to the inborn error. My young parents were completely devastated and still don't understand why it happened. The doctors told my parents it would be virtually impossible for me to ever live a "normal" life. After a month of testing I was released and today I am a thriving, happy and healthy young woman.

Throughout my childhood I experienced very few of the galactosemia-related complications that many others experience, such as speech delay and poor motor skills. I did have trouble with behavioral problems and minor learning disabilities, mainly in math.

I have been fortunate to not have experienced any major, long-term effects aside from having two cataracts. Since 1999, I have had both lenses removed and replaced with plastic lenses. Today, everything is well.

I knew nothing about galactose, whey, casein, and many other ingredients, which should be avoided. I was only told to avoid milk and milk products. I was under the impression galactosemia was rare. The doctors told my parents there was little information on the subject. Therefore, I never asked questions. I went to the genetics team to find out what galactosemia was all about because everyone was curious why I couldn't just take lactaid or some other lactose-intolerance pill. I had no answers for people who were interested.

The genetics team explained the complexities of this disease. Having spoken to several parents of galactosemic children, I was shocked at the damage this disease causes. I was completely devastated when the doctor told me the diet consisted of excluding a sugar, galactose, found in nearly every food. What worries me the most is that there are few studies on the long-term effects and what is to be expected; most importantly, if I am able to conceive.

Every person with this condition seems to be different and that makes it difficult to determine the outcome. The specialists say that POF and early menopause occur in eighty-five percent of females with galactosemia. These frightening statistics do not make it easier for me. It has been almost three years since I began a moderated diet. I feel great and thank my lucky stars every day for having all the support of others living with this disease.

I recently attended the Parents of Galactosemic Children, Inc. conference in Columbus, Ohio and have a great network of parents and other patients. I was asked to be their guest speaker at the next conference. This is the only support group for galactosemia that I have found so far. They inspired me to begin a Website to educate the public and turn this rare disorder into something positive for others living with galactosemia.

Everything I have done has proven beneficial and what I have gained is even more rewarding. Because of galactosemia, I believe I am a stronger and a better person and for that, I wouldn't trade it for the world!

It is difficult not knowing what the future holds, but I remain positive and continue to tell myself I am fertile and everything is fine. I am not certain if my ovaries are completely functional, as I had two tests done last year. One level came back too high and the second level came back too low.

The doctor did tell me I could go off the pill for one month, then get tested on the second or third day of my period. That would be the best time to get an accurate reading because I'd been on the pill for both tests. I was originally put on birth control pills at fifteen, due to irregular menstrual cycles. When I did have periods, they were erratic and infrequent. This, I was told, was no big deal because every woman's body is different.

My family doctor did not realize this could be due to galactosemia. He did not take premature ovarian failure into account. In any case, nothing was ever said to be galactosemia related. I was always told by my doctor and parents that galactosemia was a rare disease and if I eat milk products galactose would build up, causing riper cataracts and brain damage.

I was always told by my parents that, "It was just something we didn't discuss." It was who I was and not to ask anymore questions. Even though at age fifteen I wasn't sexually active, the doctor assured me that by going on the pill my menstrual cycles would return to normal. I found this a bit odd since everyone I knew went on the pill for one thing only—to prevent pregnancy.

When I moved to a different city in 1998, I met my fiancé, whose mother is a nurse. She wanted to find out exactly why I wasn't menstruating properly and why I couldn't consume milk. The only thing I could explain to her was that I had galactosemia…and I'd rather not speak about it. She found my lack of information on galactosemia unbelievable. We went to a genetics clinic to find out exactly what galactosemia was and how it was affecting my ability to eat milk and milk products.

For two and a half hours we listened to explanations about galactosemia. My blood work came back as type 1 galactosemia. I was shocked. I was shocked as to why my parents would be so embarrassed by the disease and why they would just sweep it under the carpet for all these years. More shocking was the fact that this so-called professional (my doctor), whom I had seen for more than twenty years, was so uneducated; he had put me on a birth control pill as a fifteen-year-old child and expected me to become regular, not to mention that the birth control pill he had me on contained lactose as a binding ingredient. Fortunately, after learning this, I was taken off that particular pill and put on a lactose-free pill.

You can imagine how frustrated I was and, to an extent, still am. At first, when I heard there was a high chance that galactosemia would affect my ability to conceive, it made me feel horrible and incomplete. I was letting my parents down by not providing them with all the grandchildren they often dreamed of. Most importantly, I felt as if I were alone. I was letting my fiancé and his family down for not being good enough to have many, many children. At times I feel so alone and ask myself "Why me?" After all, I was a young woman and it was only natural that my body had an urge to carry children.

In the meantime, I pray for those living with galactosemia and for those with POF and hopefully, by giving my support and strength, we can turn this into something much more positive.

May the future be brighter for those with POF. With medical advances maybe no one else will ever have to wonder, "What if?" and "Why me?"

MY LIFE'S JOURNEY

Soraya, thirty-one, diagnosed at twenty-nine

As a child I played, I dreamed, I grew. I played school. I played house. "I'm the mommy and you're the baby," I would say. I dreamed that one day I would have a family of my own.

I grew into an adolescent emotionally, physically, and mentally. I experienced friendships, good and bad. I dreamed about being a teacher and a mother. Always, throughout my dreams, there was a feeling of emptiness.

I grew into a young woman. I studied. I worked. I developed relationships. I went to college and learned about the development of children. I got engaged and married. I continued to grow as a woman, a wife, a daughter, a friend, a person. Still, something was missing, a feeling I could not understand.

Living as a married woman, I work, I study, I live and continue to change. It is a constant change in the way of thinking, of educating myself. I continue to dream. I am a woman with many dreams and desires. Dreams that do not always come true the way I wish them to. Dreams that change because of a diagnosis called POF.

Finally, a name for that emptiness: POF, undiagnosed for so many years. Wondering. Confused. Dealing with doctors who did not care and did not understand or even try to understand. Doctors who said, "You probably can't have children, but don't worry, you are still young." What did that mean? What did they know? Not much, I say! I continue to grow and change as we all do, learning about myself and POF more and more each day. It's empowering.

Living with POF, HRT, side effects and osteoporosis is a journey. Finding out what it all means takes time. Premature ovarian failure. It was such a shock to hear those words. Confusion, anger, disbelief, and mourning are all things I have and am currently going through. Finding out what hormones work for me is so hard, so confusing, because there are so many choices. Feeling empty inside—not feeling like a whole person is a terrible feeling. I feel old at twenty-nine because I have to deal with HRT and osteoporosis.

There are always challenges and struggles in life. Whether they're due to relationships, school, work, or a medical condition, everyone goes through them and comes out stronger. I feel that, in my life, I've grown in so many ways as a woman, a wife, a friend, and a POFer. I feel I am surviving and living.

Surviving POF would not have been possible without my husband, my family, my friends, especially my best friend Sonia, and of course the strength I get from God. The premature ovarian failure support group online and the local support group where I live have also been invaluable. I will continue to live, play, dream, learn, change, and grow. I will survive, and live life to its fullest. I will live out my dreams. I will be happy as I am.

MY POF STORY

Stella, twenty-seven, diagnosed at seventeen

My journey with POF began at the age of seventeen. I hadn't had a period in more than three months when I told my mother. I was sure this was just one of those things that happened. I was a senior in high school and I was under a lot of stress. Since I had begun dating the previous year my mother was deathly afraid I was pregnant. As a virgin, I assured her that was absolutely impossible.

When two weeks of progesterone failed to make me bleed, my mother's gynecologist suggested I see a reproductive endocrinologist. The RE made me very comfortable with his words, "You're obviously a focused perfectionist. I can tell that from the way you dress, your grades, and your interests (a violinist). This is no doubt stress related, but we should do some blood work."

A few days later, the doctor delivered the news to my mother on the phone. My FSH was over 120. I was in menopause and would never have biological children.

It has now been ten years since the diagnosis, and I have seen many different phases and turns this journey has to offer. From ages seventeen to twenty-one, I simply ignored POF. I was on a birth control pill like most of my friends and felt pretty normal. Heck, POF was probably just a big mistake anyway. In 1998, at twenty-two, I married my high school sweetheart, whom I had begun dating the year of my diagnosis. That's when the understanding of loss hit. I was a married woman with the responsibility of creating and caring for a family: a family I couldn't physically make.

In a way, after I married, I regressed. The thought I had at seventeen returned and boomed loud in my heart and mind. The thought was, "I have to resolve this infertility, or else." Being a religious woman, I prayed to God for a miracle. I then cursed Him with each negative pregnancy test. Two years later, when hoping became too emotionally and physically exhausting, I insisted on donor egg IVF. The day we consulted with the fertility clinic, my husband lost his job. We would have to wait. Again, I cursed God.

Those three years were emotion packed. I was angry, sad, frustrated, and honestly, I know I was depressed, too. I had stopped taking my birth control pills (unaware of the symptoms and risks) in the hope of spontaneous ovulation and was an irritable, tired, moody, depressed mess. I needed something, so I looked into POF research and found the National Institutes of Health.

At NIH, I received all the testing every POFer needs, and found that all my test results came back normal except the FSH, of course. While I was there, I saw others in much more dire situations and I became very thankful for the health I did have. Probably the best things that happened at NIH were finding the right HRT for me; an estradiol patch and Prometrium, and meeting another POFer. I felt so good on the patch—I was feeling normal again! It was enough of a turnaround that hubby and I came to a decision; we would stop thinking about babies for a year. Instead, we would focus on our marriage and find what happiness we could there.

It's amazing what perspective can do for you. While looking for the good things in our marriage, I found them! I knew I had married a great guy, but until that year, I hadn't taken the time to really marvel at how good it was. I realized that many people have kids, but lack the wealth of a healthy, loving marriage. And, while kids leave the house at eighteen (hopefully), marriage lasts a lifetime! For so long I had focused on being the abnormal one woman in ten thousand who was diagnosed so young with POF. I failed to see that I was also very special and that God had blessed me with this wonderful man at the age of sixteen. The odds of meeting one's spouse in high school and marrying five years later are also terribly abnormal—that only happens to one in thousands. In addition, the burden I had unknowingly carried (a good wife gives her husband babies) was laid to rest. I realized hubby was never as concerned about my baby making abilities as he was about winning me as his wife.

During that year, I came to several realizations. The first was that in my immature, scared rush to find a way out of the pain this diagnosis brought, I had failed to complete the statement that had become my mantra, "I have to resolve this infertility, or else." Or else what? I had assumed that life would be worthless without children, and in turn implied to my husband that a life with only him would be miserable. What would a life with just him look like? Romantic dinners, boating trips, movies at midnight…hmm, this wasn't sounding so bad. In facing my fear and challenging it head on, I found there was nothing to be afraid of, being childless was nothing to run from.

The funny thing is that when I stopped running in fear, I was finally able to look at what we lost, and mourn it. It still hurts sometimes, but for the most part I'm able to look at my life —my marriage, my faith, my friends, my talents, my character—and say thanks to POF. I'm now a strong woman, capable of handling anything life throws my way, including the adoption process we now find ourselves in. I have the wisdom of life and its gifts that many never comprehend. I have an appreciation of, and fondness for, children that comes from understanding what miracles they are. In essence, POF has become my rose-colored glasses; I see everything through that experience. Honestly, it has made my life rich.

MY QUEST FOR SUPPORT

Susan, forty-two, diagnosed at thirty-six

In 1995 I was in good health and having regular cycles. For a means of birth control, my doctor suggested that I have a tubal ligation. After my tubal ligation surgery my health changed drastically. I was not informed that one possible side effect was POF due to ovarian isolation.

Two years later, I was in grave health, so my doctor ran blood work. My FSH was ninety-two, and my LH was twenty-seven. At first I was told that I had "gone through the change of life" and was "definitely postmenopausal," then I was told that I was not postmenopausal but had POF.

I asked, "What is POF?"

"Premature ovarian failure," the doctor replied. I asked why I was not menopausal and he told me that only women over the age of forty are diagnosed as menopausal and that women under the age of forty are diagnosed with POF. For "treatment" of my POF he put me on birth control pills.

I asked my doctor if my POF condition could have been caused by the tubal ligation and he told me, no. However, a local Ob/Gyn told me that yes, it could.

I made my way to the Internet, but could not find anything about "ovarian failure." I made contact with and joined the Sans Uteri group at www.findings.net. This is a support group for women who have had hysterectomies. Although I still had my uterus I related to this group because of the surgical menopausal syndrome everyone had experienced.

The group's health concerns and postings were about treatment. My question to the group was why wasn't it publicized that tubal ligation can cause POF?

Beth Tiner, the founder of Sans Uteri, suggested that I contact Catherine Corp, as she was forming an online POF support group. I immediately contacted Catherine and joined the POF support group when it went online.

Like my experience with Sans Uteri, my experience with the POF support group was mixed. I was POF, as the other women in the group were, but the majority of the women were not POF due to ovarian isolation from tubal ligation or hysterectomy, rather POF naturally or due to other means (such as chemotherapy or radiation therapy). Many women in the POF support group were diagnosed POF in their quest to become pregnant. Some women questioned why I was there. I had children and they did not. Their health concerns and postings were about fertility and treatment. My postings asked who was post-tubal and why women are not informed that tubal ligation can cause POF. I gained a great deal of support from both groups and had a bond, yet I felt like an outsider.

I had a crash course on POF and menopause. I suffered being POF (due to ovarian isolation, also known as surgical menopause) for two years with no HRT treatment. The POF I suffered was not natural, but quite sudden and occurred quickly. I experienced hormone shock and then reverse shock when (proper) HRT treatment began. For legal reasons, I underwent a second surgery to document the cause of my POF and found answers as to why women (and the public at large) are not informed of the risk of POF before tubal ligation surgery.

In 1998, with help and support from Dr. Vikki Hufnagel, the Coalition for Post Tubal Women (CPTwomen, www.tubal.org) came to be. The coalition's goals are to educate, inform and provide accurate information to women considering tubal ligation; to educate, inform, assist, and create a supportive network for post tubal women in their quest for answers and proper follow-up care, and to bring forth the needed changes that will require women to be fully and properly informed prior to tubal ligation surgery.

When CPTwomen began in 1998, no medical or health-related Websites spoke of post tubal syndrome (PTS), much less that tubal ligation can cause POF. Information about PTS was not found in any type of information that explained tubal ligation. In the fall of 1999, the CPTwomen gained the support of the Illinois National Organization for Women, with the adoption of the Tubal Ligation Resolution, which includes "educating the public."

With help from groups such as the POF support group and Sans Uteri this information is slowly being presented to the public. Today a small handful of sites explain PTS and the POF risk and the numbers are growing. Unfortunately, the American College of Obstetricians and Gynecologists still publicly denies that tubal ligation has POF risks. It has been interesting to see our progress, but our ultimate goal is to see all women informed of the POF risk before or at the time of consent to tubal ligation, not afterwards. Someday all women will be properly informed of the POF risk from tubal ligation before their surgery.

MY STORY

Brenda, forty-three, diagnosed at thirty-four

I married at age thirty-two and shortly thereafter started having hot flashes. My periods stopped and I experienced sleep deprivation as a result of the hot flashes. I was also moody as a result of no sleep. I went to several different doctors. No one could find out what was wrong with me, though some claimed to be specialists in women's health. None tested my hormone levels. They asked if I exercised excessively—I did not; was I under stress—yes. Well, then maybe it's stress. They checked my pituitary and thyroid glands. Both were okay.

I finally went to a fertility specialist and he checked my hormone levels. I was diagnosed as being in early menopause. I then got second, third and fourth opinions. The diagnoses were the same.

I was in denial for the first couple of years and would go off hormone replacement therapy only to have the hot flashes return. It was not suggested that I have a bone density test until I changed physicians again and started seeing an Ob/Gyn specialist. It was then determined that I had already had some bone loss. I am currently being checked every year. My bone density has stabilized and I am now building bone. I am also on hormone replacement therapy, take calcium supplements and do bone building exercises three to four times a week.

This health issue created many problems in my marriage and depression and confusion in my life. I am now all right with all of this at age forty-two. I realized everything happens for a reason and I have much to give the world.

The information today is so much better than it was ten years ago for POFers. Remember to count your blessings and not your woes and everything will be all right.

NOVEMBER 6, 2001

Jennifer, twenty-six, diagnosed at twenty-four

I had my whole life planned out for as long as I could remember. I would finish college, start my career, get married and start a family. I had always dreamed of having at least two children. I love kids, and having children was something I really wanted "someday in the future when I was financially stable." Things were going as planned until November 6, 2001.

I had always had a slightly unpredictable menstrual cycle. Occasionally, I would skip a month or two, then it would come back without any problems. That seemed normal for me, so I didn't think anything of it when I didn't get my period for three months. Then it stretched to six months and I realized I should go to the doctor to make sure everything was fine. In October of 2001, I went to my Ob/Gyn for my annual exam. Everything was fine with the exam itself. He told me he was going to run some tests to determine what might be causing my lack of menstruation. He started me on a birth control pill to give me my periods back and to regulate my cycle. He mentioned possibilities of a thyroid problem or premature menopause. As soon as he said those words, "premature menopause," I had a sinking feeling. I just knew that that was my problem. I went home that day and started looking up everything I could on the Internet about premature menopause. I realized that for women my age, twenty-four, the more accurate term was premature ovarian failure. I started reading the message boards of the POF support group and the early menopause Websites, and anything else I could find.

A month later, I got home from work to find a message waiting for me from my doctor's office. My doctor wanted me to come in earlier than my scheduled appointment the following week. I had been waiting for this call. I went in on November 6, 2001 and was informed that I did, in fact, have premature ovarian failure. Even though I thought I had prepared myself for this, I had really hoped it wouldn't be true. I cried in the office as my doctor explained things to me. He told me I had an FSH level of ninety-one. In a "normal" woman, the FSH level would be under ten. I was in the postmenopausal range. I was shocked; not incredibly so, but it still hurt very badly to be told that I have only about a five to ten percent chance of having my own biological child. He went on to say that I had a very good chance of carrying a child through an egg donation process. I know he was trying to explain my options to me and to give me hope, but it was very difficult for me to hear. I was in the process of grieving the loss of my own child, the biological child that would never come to be. He wanted to run several tests to try to find out why this was happening to me. I had several vials of blood drawn and went home.

My mother called when I got home and I just started crying on the phone. She rushed over and tried to comfort me and give me hope. I know she didn't really understand what I was going through, but her support meant a lot. I told my boyfriend later that day and he was incredibly supportive. He's been amazing through this whole thing and I'm so lucky to have found him. I was pretty depressed when I found out that my eighteen-year-old cousin was pregnant. I cried for hours that night. When she had her baby around Christmas time, I could not even look at it. Seeing anything having to do with babies sent me into a state of sadness. Everywhere I went, I had reminders—commercials, baby clothes and other baby items in stores, pregnant women and babies. They were everywhere, it seemed, taunting me. I just wanted to wake up from this horrible nightmare.

I returned to my doctor's office a few weeks later to get the results of the numerous tests I had been given. Everything was normal. I think that part of my diagnosis is the most difficult for me. If there was a particular reason for this happening, it would be easier for me to accept. The fact that I am perfectly "normal" otherwise makes it that much harder. There is no medical reason why this happened and that is difficult to understand.

Over the next several months I went through bouts of mood swings. I cried for no reason and I developed very dry eyes and allergies. I think I'm in a denial state now. I am not trying to have children at this point in my life, so I don't think I realize the gravity of the situation yet. I think that once I'm ready to have kids and I am unable to naturally, then I will come to accept my situation more readily. I expect to be angry. I expect to be sad. But I am a strong woman and I know I will be able to get through this. If, by some miracle, I am able to have my own biological child that will be wonderful! If I have to use egg donation or adoption, that will be fine as well. I know I have a long and tough journey ahead of me, but I will be prepared for it by staying strong and never losing hope.

AN OPEN LETTER FROM THE HEART

Mike. Husband of POFer, Carmen.
This first appeared in the December 1997
issue of the Premature Ovarian Failure Newsletter.

W omen's infertility is a subject that has garnered a sizable share of publicity in recent years. The sight of heartbroken women unable to conceive has run the gamut from the *Wall Street Journal* to *Primetime Live*. We have heard many accounts of various procedures and protocols that many women have endured in the sometimes heartrending and elusive goal of motherhood. Yet throughout this dialogue one facet of the issue that has received little attention is the feelings and role of the affected husband. I know a little bit about this subject because, you see, I am one of those husbands.

My wife and I had been married but a short time when our long-term family plans were shattered by the news that she was experiencing premature ovarian failure. Many emotions surfaced during this trying time: sadness, anger, confusion and helplessness, just to name a few. To make matters worse, much of the medical community was still in the dark ages concerning infertility. My wife endured years of misinformed doctors and healthcare providers before a correct diagnosis of her medical condition was made.

I myself knew little of the problem. At first I didn't know what to think. Outwardly, I calmed and comforted her and told her that everything would be okay. There are always options, I told her (what those options were at the time I wasn't sure). But inwardly I was very sad. Would I never know the joy of a biological offspring? Would I never see my face in the face of a little child? This was something that was very difficult to talk about, especially with Carmen. I didn't want her to feel any worse than she already did. She blamed herself for our predicament even though she knew she wasn't responsible. There were plenty of times when I just held her and told her that these were the cards we were dealt, we just had to play them the best we could. Throughout all of this I tried to maintain an outward calm, even though at times the inner turmoil raged on.

Things changed dramatically, however, when in April of 1990 we received the wonderful news that we would become the proud parents of a baby boy. Our joy was immense when little Stephen came into our lives. His adoption was one of our proudest moments. Two years later, Alexandra added another bundle of joy to our family, also through adoption. It was during this time that the feelings associated with Carmen's infertility dimmed, but were always back there in the recesses of our minds. Several attempts with donor eggs were unsuccessful. It was on our third attempt the fantastic news came that Carmen was indeed pregnant. Nine months later Katarina Vaughn was born. It was a happy and magical day. It wasn't that long ago that a "test tube baby" made world headlines, but now it's almost routine. Both science and people's attitudes have come a long way since that very sad day when we sat in that doctor's office dazed and confused. There are occasionally times when I see that sad, faraway look in my wife's eyes and I know she's thinking, "What if?"

I, too, at times, think about how differently things may have been if she had been able to conceive naturally. But you know what? I firmly believe things happen for a reason, that there are things in this life we are not meant to understand. We have to believe we are all part of God's master plan and have to do the best that we can given our own circumstances. Stephen, Alexandra, and Katarina are the joys of our lives. We love all of them differently for their uniqueness, but the same in our hearts. As wrenching an emotional issue as infertility is, I have to believe there's always a pot of gold at the end of that rainbow. During these trying times, just remember that every time a door slams in your face, somewhere God opens another.

OPENED DOORS

Carmen, thirty-nine, diagnosed at twenty-four

It's been nearly fifteen years since I was diagnosed with premature ovarian failure. I can remember as if it were yesterday, when the door slammed shut in my face. No cure, no children, no reason as to why this was happening to me.

I spent two years with symptoms that had been explained away by my military doctors: "It's not uncommon for a woman to skip periods when you exercise or have stress." My frequent attempts to get someone to listen to me about my feeling that "something" was not right led to theories that I was a hypochondriac, and I was eventually sent to the psychologist's office.

I was stationed in Hawaii, which I enjoyed greatly and led a very active lifestyle. I met my husband, Mike, there and we dated for some time before we became engaged. It was quite romantic! In preparations for our nuptials our counselor advised us to attend premarital counseling. There Mike and I had serious discussions about what we expected from each other and our visions of family. Mike wanted a large family but I, on the other hand, was not so sure about that idea.

We had been married two months when I was told by the clinic that I needed to go immediately to Ob/Gyn at the Army medical center. A missing lab report was found and I needed to be seen right away. I called my husband and we drove together to the facility. I waited what seemed to be an eternity when finally I heard my name. I got up and stood by the desk. The doctor called my name again. I answered saying, "I'm here."

"Oh, I'm sorry…I was expecting someone much older…you're going through menopause, right?"

To this day it is still unbelievable to me that someone could be so thoughtless, and to make matters worse, tell me such news in front of the entire clinic. I was twenty-four years old when I was diagnosed.

I was very upset for some time after that day. I felt so much anger, sadness and loneliness. At one point, I attempted to make my husband leave me so he could find a new wife who would give him the many children he wanted. My husband realized what I was doing. On one particularly hard day he looked me in the eyes and said, "I didn't marry you for your ability to have children. I married you because I love you. We can still be parents in other ways."

I will never have a biological child. The winds of fate closed that door. It was in a sense a death of the child that never will be, and I grieved. Strangely enough, I never felt any other loss. Some women I have met have felt a loss of their womanhood, a loss in becoming less than a person. I never based my self-worth on whether or not I could have children. Honestly, I had never given it much thought.

The door opened on April 24, 1990, when a young woman entered the room with a most beautiful baby boy. The adoption social worker stood there as she introduced us to our new son who was only nineteen days old. His birth mother handed him to me and we both stared at him, hugged and cried. It was the most wonderful day of my life, aside from getting married that is.

We are now parents of four children: three adopted and one by donor IVF. I am Mommy in every sense of the word—cook, maid, taxi driver and nurse. My husband and I have fostered seven children to date, as well. POF may have closed some of our options, but it didn't stop us from fulfilling our desire to be parents. POF never goes away. We still have to worry about taking better care of ourselves, but, it most definitely is not the worst disorder to have. We can still live happy and healthy lives, and for this I am grateful.

THE PILL

Emma, twenty-nine, diagnosed at eighteen

On December 9, 1987 I wrote in my journal, "Thank you God, for making me normal!" I was thirteen and too shy to write that I'd had my first period that day.

Months later I would go back to that entry and cross out that sentence. In fact, I'd be furious at God for making me different. But on that December 9, something else happened that I was unprepared for.

"You're a woman! Emma, my precious bean! My darling! You're all grown up now!" My mother couldn't help being so overcome. I felt a bit angry with her though. This was my body, not hers! I was glad to be a woman, but I wanted some privacy. Wasn't that part of the bargain of growing up?

I was so disturbed by my mother's fuss over the New Me that I was glad my period didn't come back the following month. My mother asked me if I'd had another one. "No," I said.

"Not to worry," she replied. "Sometimes it's like that."

During the next few months, my period didn't come back. But I was fourteen. Some girls started late, I knew. Maybe it hadn't been a period after all. I wondered, maybe my hymen had broken. I had no idea what a hymen was, but I had read somewhere that if it broke, it could mimic a period.

In December 1988 I visited my father and stepmother in Canada and it occurred to me that I could move there to live with them. When I went back to England I told my mother I was leaving.

Some time during the next six months my mother hauled me in front of a doctor to have me tell him my periods were nonexistent. Out of embarrassment, I lied and said I had had more than one. At least that's what my mother says now. I remember seeing a doctor, having blood drawn, and being asked about strange stretch marks on my body. I don't remember him asking about periods.

The doctor called my mother to say there was a problem with the results; there was a mistake and the tests had to be run again. By now, however it was summer 1989, and everything was in place for my move to Canada. There was no time to go to the doctor to follow up. I left England in June 1989.

That summer my dad, stepmother and I hunted for a house in a good neighborhood in Toronto. September was exciting and scary with new classes, new friends, a new house, and a new family. My stepmother asked me about my periods, but there was nothing to talk about. I still hadn't started. Anyway, I was well-developed otherwise, so we figured they'd show up eventually.

When the school year ended, I went on a road trip across Canada with my stepmother and a friend of hers. On the prairies we stopped at a public washroom and I was horrified to see blood in my underwear. Lots of it! I came out and sheepishly told my stepmother.

"Do we need to stop for supplies?" she asked.

"No," I said. "It'll go away."

She took me at my word, and we kept driving.

When we woke up the next day in a motel in the Rocky Mountains, I had a new constellation of zits on my forehead and more blood in my underwear. Lovely! I wasn't happy, and my stepmother wasn't pleased either, as we had to find an open drugstore in this sleepy town—on a Sunday! Luckily the Kmart was open.

After that I watched and waited for another menstrual ambush, but none came.

I was glad to get it again, but uneasy when I thought about it. Deep down I felt I had made it go away just by hating it so much. Still, as the months passed I felt less afraid of it and more hopeful it would come back. Besides, this didn't seem to be so normal. By now I was sixteen.

When I was seventeen, the doctor ran blood tests and noticed some strange results. She said it was probably nothing to be concerned about, but she wanted me to take a drug, Provera, for a few weeks to see if I would have a period on that. There were no side effects, she said. If I didn't have a period, I was to get back in touch with her. Since I was going to university the next day, I wouldn't see her again for a few months, but she said I'd probably have "a bleed" anyway so it wouldn't be a problem. I wasn't sure what she meant, but I took the Provera anyway. No period arrived.

In my first year of classes I sometimes had the strangest sensations. Monday, Wednesday and Friday mornings I had English at nine o'clock. Outside it was minus twenty Celsius and I'd dress in a big heavy sweater to cross the courtyard from residence to class. Ten minutes into class, my face would flush and I'd have to take off all the layers of clothing I had, down to my T-shirt. I felt like I was melting! Then there were nights when I'd be dropping off to sleep only to wake up covered in sweat.

I saw my doctor again while I was home for Christmas. She told me that my blood tests, the hot flashes, and the Provera meant I was in "premature menopause." Menopause? Yes indeed! I could never have children. Never? Well, maybe some scientific advancements would enable me to have children, but it was unlikely. To prevent osteoporosis—brittle bones and fractures—by the time I was in my twenties, she said I should take birth control pills.

The pill?

Yes. The pill contained a form of the hormone needed to prevent osteoporosis. The only thing was, I needed to use other contraception if I was to become sexually active, because although I would probably never have children, there was a chance I might.

This sounded so crazy to me that I almost laughed out loud. She wanted me to take the pill because I couldn't have kids, but use contraception... because maybe I *could*?

At eighteen I was an avid Greenpeace supporter. My best friend was on an anti-Candida diet to combat allergies to citric acid and caffeine. My mother was a promoter of homeopathic remedies for everything and my father was a keen proponent of the benefits of exercise and fresh air. I was a vegetarian, a teetotaler, a nonsmoker—I didn't even drink coffee. I was not ready to take ANY drugs, prescription or no!

Havoc reigned in my family. My mother cried every day and told me the doctors had to be wrong. She said I should see a homeopath, a naturopath, change my diet—it couldn't be menopause. I became increasingly angry with her. I felt she was ignoring what was wrong. The blood tests showed I had this. There was no turning back, no fixing this.

Yet I didn't want to take the pill. Even my doctor said there was a link between taking estrogens and breast cancer. Why risk it?

My father was angry when I said I didn't want to go on the pill, yet when I pointed out the risk of breast cancer, he had no answers. He was frustrated and worried about me, but didn't know what to say.

My compromise was to wait until the end of first year, May 1992, before going on the pill. in May I began taking a low-dose pill called LoEstrin.

For the next few years it was as if this hadn't happened. I was pleased I could have my periods come or go at will. When I felt like it, I was just another woman, with cramps, headaches, and all. I knew, or thought I knew, there was a risk of breast cancer, but I preferred not to think about it. Besides, the doctors hadn't said it was impossible to have children, just extremely unlikely. What did they know, anyway? When had they ever been able to explain why this had happened to me?

I figured I'd pass on contraception. If I were to get pregnant then, well, I'd just drop everything and have a baby. If it were my only chance it would have to be basically an act of God.

Ten years passed. Then, during the summer of 2002, the Women's

Health Initiative (WHI) held a press conference to say they were canceling a study because it showed the link between estrogen replacement and breast cancer. The day I read that article was the last day I took the pill.

I discovered a research project on POF going on at the National Institutes of Health in the United States. I was lucky enough to be admitted there as a subject for their research. A week after I returned from NIH I went on the form of hormone replacement therapy they recommend. The staff at NIH informed me that women with POF have a far lower risk of breast cancer, all things being equal. By taking estrogen every day we essentially raise our risk up to the "normal" one faced by everyone. That's not quite as scary as I had originally imagined.

A nurse friend once asked me how I felt on the birth control pill. She said it gave her a "flat affect."

"Huh," I said. "What's that?"

"When you don't feel anything," she replied.

I was quiet, wondering what it was like to feel strong emotions anyway. People had often commented that I tended to be detached and unemotional. For years that conversation stayed with me.

Since I've started the HRT recommended at NIH I take a cyclical dose of estrogen and progesterone, It is the first time I have had estrogen in my body without added progesterone. I guess it's true what they say; estrogen effects your mood! I have experienced a peace of mind and well-being that I used to feel only occasionally. It occurs to me that I've been going around for years with a "flat affect" and mild depression caused by the pill. Progesterone is famous for its PMS symptoms. Imagine having mild PMS every day for ten years! That's what it's like for some women on the pill.

I'm not a doctor and I'm not an expert on POF or HRT. Young women like me are supposed to take more estrogen, so the theory goes, because they need more to protect their bones. Still, that's no reason to automatically feed them the pill. There are enough varieties and strengths of HRT out there to meet unique needs. You don't even have to limit yourself to brand name drugs. There's something called a compounding pharmacy that will make up the strength that is right for you.

New HRT doesn't change life without children, however. That takes a lot longer to get used to. To all those with POF out there, I wish you luck on this long, interesting journey.

POF—THE JOURNEY
NEVER ENDS

Suzanne, thirty-eight, diagnosed at twenty

It all started back in 1986 when I became aware that something just wasn't quite right. I was twenty and in March of that year I got the news. I was living in Los Angeles and pursuing my dreams of being an entertainer. I had no boyfriend and no thoughts whatsoever of marriage or children. If I had only understood what a life-altering diagnosis it was, I do believe I would have made other choices.

I was a late developer. My menses started when I was almost seventeen. I had hot flashes starting at age eighteen. I was going to Planned Parenthood for my gynecological care and in 1985 went for a regular checkup. I took the pill and it made me feel like someone had injected water just under the surface of my skin. After two months, I chose a diaphragm instead. That was July 1985, and I have never had a natural period since. In October, I visited an Ob/Gyn who ran blood tests and said I was fine.

After eight months with no period, my mother obtained a referral for me from her Ob/Gyn. In March of 1986, I made an appointment with the referred doctor, a reproductive endocrinologist (RE). He asked for a copy of the tests done the previous October, so I obliged. The RE didn't even examine me or take one test. I came into his office and he reviewed the blood test results. He then wrote on my chart those three magic letters that have forever changed my life: POF. Clearly, the previous doctor did not know how to interpret the same results! This was my first lesson in realizing how many doctors do not understand or know about POF. I was one of the lucky ones; everything was kindly and carefully explained to me. I was offered counseling if I was upset. Everyone wanted me to be upset. I remember thinking, "Should I be upset? I don't have to worry about birth control and I don't ever see myself as a parent anyway." This was good news to me.

Life went on. I slowly learned to accept that I would have to take a pill every day for the rest of my life. That was the hardest thing for me. Just before my twenty-second birthday, I met my future ex-husband. We dated for three months and it was at that point that I realized I had the responsibility to tell him what he was in for if we were to get serious. I prayed and kept asking for guidance as to when to talk to him. One night, I suddenly had the feeling that this was the moment. I remember feeling extremely vulnerable and damaged as I quietly explained to him what POF was. I told him that if he wanted a life with children, I was not the woman for him. He said I was enough for him and he did not need children in his life. At the time, I was told I had a twenty-five percent chance of spontaneous ovulation, so we agreed to forego all forms of birth control and let fate take control. I somehow just knew it would never happen.

A year later, my depression kicked in. After a year of therapy, I was stamped "clinically depressed" and sent to a psychiatrist. I was put on an antidepressant. I took that along with Premarin and Provera for approximately eight years. The antidepressant got me out of my fog and enabled me to live my life. I tried several times over the years to go off of it, but the deep bouts with anger would come back with a vengeance, so I knew I was not ready. What I didn't understand until later was that Provera was responsible for my depression. This was my lesson in how some doctors like to give people a pill to fix a pill.

Around the age of thirty a lot started happening. I was an office manager and a married homeowner by now (although a rock singer by night). My marriage wasn't going well and I decided to leave my husband. By this time, I had successfully taken myself off the antidepressant. I felt the need to see what life was like without it again and I have not felt the need for it since. I had also changed my progesterone as well.

By October 1998, I was again not feeling well. I discovered the beginnings of severe melasma and felt Premarin had everything to do with it. Coincidentally, I ran across an article on Premarin horses. I was astonished at how Premarin is made and what torture pregnant horses go through to make this medication (PRE=pregnant, MAR=mare, IN=urine). All I could think of was that I needed to stop supporting this practice and I had to change my medication immediately. It was then that I took the leap into the estradiol (bioidentical estrogen) patch (Premarin is conjugated estrogen). This was the beginning of possibly the most painful episode of all my POF problems. I switched to the patch, along with Prometrium. What I didn't know at the time was that my body had never produced standard levels of estradiol, so getting a normal dose all at once was clearly too much.

By Thanksgiving, I was crying every morning as my huge, water-filled breasts adjusted to gravity. I was twenty pounds overweight, my hair was falling out and I had developed cystic acne on my face and scalp! My New Year's resolution for 1999 was to get healthy no matter what it took. I went on a major diet in February and changed to a lower dose patch in March. My hair had started to grow back and the weight was coming off slowly but my breasts still hurt terribly and the cystic acne persisted.

I was still not feeling great and I decided I needed to investigate. One day I typed "POF" into the search engine of my computer at work. Lo and behold the POF support group Website came up. It actually was in its infancy then. At last people who understood me! As I started to read the stories, I was again shocked to learn about many people's experiences, including those with depression in relation to prolonged Provera use. I also learned about osteoporosis for the first time and the bone density test. I came to the conclusion that I had not been given all the facts about even more things and I was angry. I demanded to get off the patches and sadly went back to Premarin. I chose to stay with Prometrium due to what I had found out about Provera and its connections to depression. By June I had lost fifteen pounds and I was feeling more like myself again.

Ten years into POF and it was already too late to prevent my then-borderline osteopenia, the precursor to osteoporosis. Today I have osteopenia and work every day to combat the onset of osteoporosis with calcium supplements, exercise and medication. Along with my bone test, I also had my first mammogram. My doctor thought she felt a lump and I was so frightened. After an ultrasound and mammogram it was determined that there was no lump, but my breast tissue density was massive. I now get a mammogram every year. Also, we made plans for me to stay on Prometrium, then the next year start to explore other forms of estrogen. I thought it was a reasonable plan. When I called to make my appointment the next year, the doctor had left the practice with no notice to her patients.

I was left high and dry. Again I turned to the POF Website. There was a local RE listed and I made an appointment with her. I listened as she explained my condition to a nurse she was training. I thought, here is a doctor who truly "gets it." I explained to her my feelings about Premarin and my horrific experience with the patch. I was very specific that I did not want anything like those medications. What I did not realize was that she had stopped listening. She launched into what I affectionately call "the speech" as she started my pelvic exam. "The speech" is when a doctor launches into all the alternative methods for having children and gives me the latest data on success rates, etc. I calmly stopped her and explained that I found it hard enough to deal with my health every day and I did not have any interest in ever pursuing pregnancy or parenthood. What I didn't know was that she made her living primarily from egg donation procedures. She had one protocol of

116

treatment: for patients who wanted to be parents. That wasn't me. She refused to ever see me again and did not even assist in a referral. Yet another lesson was learned: not all REs want to work with POF patients who do not want to get pregnant. It is very important to find that out before you make an appointment.

It's amazing, though, how at the darkest times in life God can set you on the right path with the assistance of our angels right here on earth. I had been corresponding via email for about a year with a fellow POFer from the Website. It was at this point that she suggested I think about going to the National Institutes of Health (NIH) and participate in the protocol screening for POF research with her. After all, they are the experts and maybe they could give me the information I needed to take care of myself. I had known about the studies, but thought going to Maryland was too much of a bother and expense. However, this time it sounded right. We ended up going together and she and I have remained very good friends.

My experience at the NIH is another story altogether, but for me it was important and I am glad I experienced it. I can only hope that my participation will help others who are and will be struggling with POF in the future. I have since received some valuable information from the NIH. I have chosen to pursue a homeopathic course of treatment in my never-ending attempt for hormonal harmony with my body and spirit.

Currently, I am diagnosed with POF, Hashimoto's thyroiditis and osteopenia. No happy ending to this story, but I continue to hope for a better day and some sort of balance to my health. I, of course, couldn't get through my daily struggles without the love and support of my significant other, family and friends. May we all continue to strive for a better life through whatever means possible and above all, my fellow POFers—never give up!

PREPARING FOR INJECTIONS

This appeared as a question with responses on the POFSG listserv

Hi everyone,

I went to my RE today for injection "lessons." When I left, I started crying. I feel so stupid for crying, but I think I am afraid that if this doesn't work, I am going to feel really let down. Has anyone else experienced these kinds of emotions prior to starting infertility treatments?

By the way, I am on BCPs right now, and once I have a period, I am going on Gonal-F (eight ampules), followed up with progesterone.

Best,
Jennifer

Hi Jennifer,

You are definitely not alone on this one! I am deathly afraid of going through this. I'm going on a new insurance that pays for IVF in January and will be starting my first cycle in March. As we get closer and closer, I get more and more nervous about the injections. It's very scary and all sounds to me like something a trained medical professional should be doing instead of me and my husband!

I'm also just getting to the stage where I'm thinking about what my emotional state will be if the treatments don't work. For the most part I've just been dreading the process itself and now it's starting to sink in that the process really isn't guaranteed and I may go through all this for nothing.

Please continue to share your experience. It will help people like me know what to expect!

Vicki

Jennifer,

I have to say that crying seems like a good response to starting an IVF cycle. I went through one and really, my emotions were all over the map. The battle between hope and preparing oneself for disappointment is wrenching. Of course you'll feel let down if it doesn't work! It makes perfect sense. You're very brave for going through all this. Books and books have been written about the emotional roller coaster of IVF. Some feel pressure to try procedures they don't really want, because the end justifies the means. Others don't realize the toll that all the procedures will take on them, emotionally. But you know, POF is tough. You've gone through that, you're going through that, and you're dealing with it as best you can. One "problem" with all the infertility treatments, wonderful though they are, is that they give you the illusion of control over your fate. There's the illusion that you have some control over whether or not you have children, so if the IVF doesn't work, you've done something wrong—or dealing with infertility and accepting it is delayed. I wish you the best of luck in this procedure! It could work, it might not. One wise word I had from someone who had been through the infertility wrencher was how wonderful adoption was. They knew that at the end of the process, they would have a child through adoption, whereas there's no guarantee with IVF. For the next few months, you'll be in a limbo of waiting. Just try to take care of yourself as best you can during that time!

Also, to Vicki,

Frankly, I was surprised at how easy it is to inject yourself, and to mix all the things that need mixing (Gonal-F and water, for example), measure the things that need measuring, etc. It's really not for very long, either. Just a few weeks. These are subcutaneous injections, by the way. The intramuscular injections are trickier, but I don't think you'll need to do them, except for the HCG.

Once when I was younger, I tried to stick myself with a needle to get some blood for an experiment, and found that it was really hard to do. But my feelings about the IVF were so positive, I felt that it could be a good thing, that I really didn't think about any difficulty with sticking a needle into me and it was easy to do. There isn't really any pain, either. You can barely feel it. There is a film that Serono Pharmaceuticals will send you with your Gonal-F, showing you exactly how to do it, too.

As for going through it for nothing: Fortunately for you, your financial investment is small. You can think about it as a way of making sure you did all you could to try to get pregnant. That way, even if it doesn't result in a pregnancy, you can say, "Well, at least I tried." So it won't be for "nothing."

Take care,
Gillian

THE SECOND ACT

Lisa, forty-three, diagnosed at thirty-nine

I remember the leaves. Bright, crisp leaves blowing through the air, landing with grace on the surface they choose. I felt very small as I walked to my car, trying to digest the news the doctor had given me. Menopause. A word that held no significance in my life. A word that conjured up images of gray-haired ladies, sipping tea and discussing their ailments as their grandchildren played outside. Dear God, this could not be happening to me! It must be a mistake. I'm only thirty-nine.

When I think back to that dreary day in November when life took me on a journey I could not foresee, I still feel a sense of loss; The loss of a carefree child who shared a body with the woman I had become, without me even realizing it.

I was diagnosed with endometriosis when I was thirty. The diagnosis itself gave me a feeling of relief, after struggling with my body through excruciating periods for the previous five years. I tried all the medicinal approaches, from birth control pills to Lupron injections—all to no avail. Relief from the pain and heavy periods was a hiatus that was too short-lived.

Well into my thirties, and five laparoscopies later, I decided that a hysterectomy was my only answer. At thirty-eight the decision was made. It was a decision I felt at peace with. My sense of well-being, and a renewed exuberance for life, grew in those months following my surgery. The pain was gone and all things seemed possible. The world was my oyster...then it began.

Nine months after my surgery I began to feel subtle changes in my body. A body once quite predictable was now sending me messages I didn't quite understand. I would occasionally wake up drenched in sweat, my night clothes clinging to me, when the room temperature was only sixty-eight degrees. The hot flashes that followed would always catch me off-guard, and I'd find myself removing clothing as the perspiration trickled down my face. Insomnia, joint pain, and a libido that was taking me on a roller coaster ride were all players in a diagnosis that was about to shake the very foundation of my being.

I wasn't passive about the changes going on in my body, just ignorant of the over all picture. I went to an orthopedic surgeon for the hip pain that prevented me from sleeping, and a urologist for the occasional water retention. I developed a twitch in my left eye, so off I went to an ophthalmologist who told me I was in need of reading glasses. I finally went to my primary physician, who did an LH, FSH, and estradiol profile. The results were devastating. Postmenopausal. Those were the words that echoed through me as I walked to my car with my estrogen patch in one hand and my blood work results in another. I sat in my car as tears fell upon the report that designated my fate, blurring each number that represented a new phase in my life.

After the initial shock wore off and my estrogen patch was securely in place, I began to reassess my life. The brain-fog decreased and my sense of reasoning slowly returned. I began to devour every book I could possibly find on premature ovarian failure. I surfed the Web for all relevant articles and created a folder for future reference. I started researching the various forms of treatment and how they might benefit me. Osteoporosis and heart disease were illnesses that had no personal meaning to me until now.

I felt a growing empowerment within me. Instead of fighting the occasional hot flash or night sweat, I began to float with it, to experience the full impact of the message I was being sent. The estrogen I was taking surged through me like a delicious elixir, revitalizing my organs and bringing my mind back to clarity. I started to embrace the metamorphosis I was going through and, in doing so, developed a more definite sense of who I was as a woman. Menopause did not have to mean the end of my femininity and sexuality, but rather the beginning of a new journey into a better understanding of myself.

If my life were a play, this would be the second act. The act in which the true substance of the characters is explored. A time of rebirth and discovery. A time that precedes the third act...when the final curtain falls.

So It Starts

Steph, nineteen, told of diagnosis at twelve

There I was, twelve years old, and everything up to then had been okay. I'd had my first two holidays abroad and was happy at home. School was the same and I had loads of normal friends. I was verging on the start of puberty. In our gym class all the girls were given a sanitary towel, tampon and sex talk. Everyone was so embarrassed and we all just laughed. We were all given big samples of towels and tampons to take home.

Later that night my mum seemed a bit weird when I showed her the stuff, but I figured it was because I was her first child and I was growing up. I went to my room and hid them in my knicker drawer. I was so glad and felt so grown up that I had them because I was starting to think I would never have a period, but now I knew it was nearly here. Then my mum came into my room with tears in her eyes. I asked what was wrong and she said she had something she had to tell me.

First off, I thought she was going to tell me she has AIDS! Around that time in the UK there was a TV program about a guy with AIDS and it was horrible, and I figured it had to be something bad for her to be crying.

Then she told me I wouldn't be having periods like other girls and wouldn't be able to have children. That blew me away. She said it was because I was born without a womb and ovaries. I thought this was weird because I had everything else like a normal girl (boobs coming on and a vagina). Apparently no one knew apart from me, my mum and my dad. My dad didn't live with me, so he wasn't there.

This tore me apart inside. I went to school the next day and couldn't concentrate. I hadn't cried until this point, not until I started to think about how I had played with dolls when I was little and how I thought I would have a little girl and name her India when I grew up. I felt as if everything I had known was a sham and that the previous twelve years of my life had been a lie. Not that my mum had lied, but everything I had dreamed and thought would happen to me was no longer going to happen. I was off school for a week. My mum couldn't deal with it all that well. She found it hard to talk without getting really upset.

I told my best friend just after that and she turned to me and said, "Does that mean you are a lesbian?" I was so shocked by this I decided not to tell anyone else.

My mum told me that I had to see a doctor now that I knew, as I had a minor surgery to undergo. The day we went to see the doctor I felt strange. That was because we went to the hospital we had gone to for years about my hernia operation. My mom then told me the truth.

When I was two weeks old my aunt discovered a hernia in my stomach. We went to the hospital and I had my operation. During the operation they found I had no womb or anything inside. Dad was distraught, blaming himself, and Mum was dumbfounded. Every year since I had gone to this hospital and had a checkup on my stomach for what I thought was my hernia operation. I always spoke to the doc and had an abdominal examination. Then I would sit outside and my mum would talk to the doctor for a while. She always came out crying and I didn't know why. I thought it was because she remembered when I was little and I had to have an operation.

Now that I knew it felt totally different when I went to see the doc. He talked more about the condition I had. This was the moment I found out I had androgen insensitivity syndrome (AIS). He explained that I had no womb because I had XY chromosomes like a boy. A fault on the X chromosome meant it didn't fully develop so I was a girl, but none of my reproductive organs had developed. He also told me that I had two small tissues in my lower abdomen which were known as dormant testes. Alarms bells are ringing at this point! Am I a boy? What the hell is going on?

He tells me I have to have an operation to remove these.

From that point until my operation when I was fourteen I had to take birth control pills for estrogen and progesterone as I didn't have any of my own. This was a daily reminder of my AIS.

When I had my operation I was in hospital for two days. I had an epidural so I couldn't feel a thing, but it was so painful when that wore off. I was off school for six weeks and could hardly walk.

After that I still had to take my pill, but it was okay because I thought everything had been done and I could get on with my life. I spoke too soon.

I grew up after that as a normal teenage girl and had the normal experiences: boys, alcohol (don't tell my mum). When I was nearly sixteen I had my first sexual experience. What a nightmare! I bled all over. I knew girls bled, but mine was like a river. I brushed it off. I started to see a gynaecologist every six months to get my pill, but by this point I was more curious so she referred me to a special gynecologist consultant. I was seventeen and wanted to know more. He told me that AIS girls sometimes don't develop a full vagina. It can be no more that a dimple. After several internal exams we discovered that my vagina was half the size of a normal vagina. I was disappointed, but thought it was better than nothing.

By this time I was taking high doses of Prozac. I was suffering from suspected manic depression due to my AIS. I hated myself, was ashamed and had no self-esteem. I felt I couldn't live and had several suicide plans.

Then I went to an AISSG meeting. I met lots of girls with AIS and found out a lot more about my condition. It enlightened me and made me feel less alone. Still, my feelings didn't stop. I had recurring bouts of depression that wouldn't go away.

While I was at the meeting a girl told me of a surgery she had undergone which lengthened her vagina. It was called a partial colo-vaginoplasty. I discussed this with my doc and he told me what the surgery was about. They take part of your colon and attach it to your vagina to lengthen it. I was sold. By this time I had had a few serious boyfriends and knew that sex wasn't enjoyable and thought this was my meal ticket to a better sexual experience.

I was off work for three months. I was in hospital for two weeks with no food or drink. I was on a morphine drip, I was spaced out all of the time. The first operation was painful, but this as far worse. I had friends around me all of the time, which made me better, and my family showed so much support.

Within no time I was back to work and feeling great.

I am now nineteen and it's been eight months since my operation. I am off the antidepressants and feel much better. I have a normal life—fights with mum, job worries. I am functioning like a normal young girl.

I have had sex since the operation and it is a marked improvement.

I have just done an interview with *Marie Claire UK* magazine and hope this brings enlightenment to people about a subject which is seen by most as taboo.

SOMETIMES

Kris, thirty-three, diagnosed at twenty-nine

Sometimes I wish there was a cure
So I wouldn't have to think anymore

Sometimes I feel I'm not the same
Even though I know there's nothing to blame

Sometimes it's just too much to take
And I beseech my mind to take a break

Sometimes there is nowhere to go
And I never thought I could get so low

Sometimes I don't know what to do
And it seems that nobody has a clue

Sometimes I wonder what would be
If I didn't have to worry for me

Sometimes I feel I can't go on
But I would miss too much if I were gone

There Isn't Enough Soy in the World

Caryn, thirty-five, diagnosed at twenty-four

It took only a couple of doctors a couple of years to determine my diagnosis of premature ovarian failure at age twenty-four. Many women are not that lucky. I immediately started having irregular periods at the onset of my menstruation at age sixteen. By the time I was twenty-one they were almost nonexistent. When I became sexually active I went on birth control pills, which hid most of my symptoms. When I went off the pill, I didn't get my period and I experienced hot flashes at twenty-two. Doctors began to run tests; I had normal thyroid readings, normal chromosomal information, but a very high follicle stimulating hormone level—one of the indicators of POF.

During this time, I was in college and had met my husband. We were together two years when I was diagnosed with POF. We were married two years later, determined to deal with the issues of our fertility when the time came. By the time we started trying to get pregnant, I had been off the pill for two months and had horrible hot flashes and a FSH reading of 126. I was trying to regulate my low estrogen level with a lot of soy products. My doctor said, "There isn't enough soy in the world..." and put me on hormone replacement therapy consisting of two milligrams of estrogen daily with ten days of progesterone per month. We even tried one round of injections, but stopped after three days when my ovaries showed no response to the shots.

Six months later, we were at a Resolve conference and had decided to look into the adoption process when we found out we were six weeks pregnant with our daughter Anna. We had only tried for a year to get pregnant. I took progesterone for the first trimester and had a textbook pregnancy and delivery. I was even able to breast feed for about six months until my milk dried up and my hot flashes came back. I went back on HRT and we started trying again. We were thrilled and amazed only two years later to find out we were pregnant again with what looked like another healthy fetus. At sixteen weeks we were devastated when there was no heartbeat.

Our daughter, Anna, is three years old now and for the past year we have been trying to get pregnant again, without success. We are trying a round of shots to try to stimulate ovulation. I'm hopeful and doubtful.

The past year has brought a lot of soul searching. What are we willing to do in order to expand our family? How do we treat my POF in light of current findings about HRT, my symptoms, and our desire for another child? How has our infertility and our loss affected our self-esteem, our relationships, and our marriage? And, of course, there is a precious, wonderful child at home who needs us in the midst of our turmoil and pain. It has been a difficult year.

I often wish for the future when our family building and some of these questions will be behind us. My mother is quick to point out though, that every decade brings with it its own issues. This is true, I am sure. My journey is teaching me to have a tremendous amount of patience and is calling on my every last reserve of strength. I have found healing, comfort and hope in reaching out to the POF support group that is helping us POFers to not feel so alone and to find strength in each other and in our stories.

You'll Have Babies, the Doctors Are Wrong

June, thirty, diagnosed at twenty-two

"You'll have babies, the doctors are wrong." These are the words I hear every time I bring up my POF with a family member or friend. It's as though they have it and are trying to avoid it. Every time I hear those words it's as though a dagger is thrust into my heart. Because of these words I can't talk with anyone about POF and therefore have had to deal with it internally, which in several instances almost cost me my life. I hope that by relating my story I can help others who also have to deal with this situation on their own.

I was twenty-two when I was diagnosed with POF. Until then, I never wanted to have children. In fact, on any given day you could hear me say something like, "I never want to have any children." or "I love children, as long as they're not mine."

Who knew that one day I'd be eating those words? In college I had two abortions because my career and my independence were more important to me than a human life. Every single day, I ask if God decided to take all my kids away from me because I took away two of his.

At first diagnosis, POF wasn't a big deal to me. I wasn't menstruating anymore, which, to me, was a big plus. I wasn't thinking about marriage and children because I was too young. "POF, it's no big deal," I said to myself. I never talked about it or even thought about it. Close friends didn't even know I had it until three years later.

Three years later, at twenty-five my spiral to hell began. I remember sitting at dinner with some friends and we were discussing getting married and having children. We were at that age when we wanted to settle down and start having families. Two of us out of our circle of five had just gotten engaged. Career-wise, we were all doing well and now we wanted to share our lives with one special person. This is when it dawned on me that I couldn't have any children. The rest of that night my mood was somber. I made sure to keep my wineglass full so that I could drown myself in alcohol and not think about it. I could feel my body wanting to get up and walk out of the restaurant. From that moment on, everything in the restaurant became one big blur; the people, the conversation lost focus. I became lost in my thoughts. I wanted to go home and feel sorry for myself.

On my way home that night, sitting on the train alone, it hit me again. I couldn't have any children. At that instant, I obtained a second voice in my head that would remind me of this fact every single day. It was like my head became haunted by an evil spirit. Every time I looked at a man and thought he was attractive, this evil voice would say, "What are you looking at that guy for? Once he finds out you can't have any kids he won't want you." My goodness, this voice is right. What am I going to do? I'll be single forever. I'm damaged goods. No man would want me. The battle in my head became more and more intense as the weeks went by and my mental health secretly deteriorated.

The only way I knew how to control this voice was by drinking. I'd drink every night when I returned home from work. I was living with my parents, so I'd lock myself in my room and get out the big bottle of vodka I kept hidden in my closet. Drinking made the voice go away temporarily. I knew I needed help, but as an African-American woman, I was taught to deal with my own problems and not let others know my personal business.

Attempting to ignore that belief, I picked up the phone one night and told a close friend of my POF diagnosis. The conversation was weird. She was shocked and didn't know what to say. She told me that the doctors were wrong and I'd have lots of kids. She was the first of many to make that statement. In order to lighten up this uncomfortable ordeal, I made little remarks referring to me not wanting to have any children anyway; at least I'd be able to keep my great figure. We laughed and changed the subject. I got off the phone, poured a glass of vodka, and went to sleep. My friend's reaction convinced this was something I had to keep to myself.

A month later I moved to San Francisco to live with a friend. At this point, I was dying inside and didn't know what else to do. The evil voice in my head got progressively worse, and I couldn't keep a decent relationship with a man for fear that once he found out I couldn't have kids, he'd leave. I made sure not to get emotionally attached to anyone. I guess I thought that if I left New York, the voice, the drinking, and the depression would all stay behind. They didn't. A year later I was back in New York. It's true what they say about not being able to run away from your problems.

I returned home, but I was still in bad shape. By this time a few more friends knew about my POF because I would mention it in passing. I made sure to make it sound as though I could care less about having kids. They told me the doctors were lying. I'd have lots of kids. I was dying with each and every breath I took. My depression led to three suicide attempts. Attempt number one happened one night after a friend told me she was pregnant. That evil voice in my head went to work, loud as ever, telling me how worthless I was. I didn't feel attractive and I had convinced myself that I'd be alone forever. I decided that since I was going to be alone for the rest of my life I wanted to die, but a combination of vodka and four or five sleeping pills didn't do the trick. I woke up the next morning sick as ever. I was in bad shape and couldn't go to work. Obviously, the next two attempts failed as well. I stopped trying to end my life.

When I turned twenty-seven. I was still depressed, trying to keep everything to myself. I was barely making it through life. Each day was an effort to get out of bed. My menopause symptoms were bad. I attempted to have a relationship but it failed because I wouldn't get close. Funny, I tell this man about my POF and he hugged me. He told me he loved me no matter what and he would always be with me. Then he said, "What do doctors know? You'll have lots of kids one day." Why wouldn't people stop saying that? Did they learn that from a book entitled, *What To Say To A Friend With POF*? Our relationship ended.

At twenty-eight, after failed suicide attempts, relationships gone bad, drinking every night, and depression, I decided to stop feeling sorry for myself and try to make it through this thing. After all, I would be dealing with it for the rest of my life. I told myself that everything happens for a reason. If God chose not to allow me to have children, maybe there was a good reason behind it. I could always adopt, and if a man left me because of my POF, then he wasn't meant for me.

There's so much I could tell you about how POF has affected my life, but I'd need more than these pages. I could tell you things like how happy I was when a friend miscarried because for a moment I figured well, if she can't have kids then I'm not alone anymore. We could wallow in sorrow together. I regret feeling that today.

Today my thinking is more positive, something that didn't happen overnight. In fact, I'm still depressed at times and that evil voice is still there. However, instead of forcing it away with alcohol, I force it away with positive thoughts. I definitely need outside help, but until I can afford it I'm just taking things day by day. All I can tell someone with POF is that it's not the end of the world. Don't do what I did and treat it that way. Talk to people, that's the most important thing to do, and know that you're beautiful.

WILL I EVER BE A MOM?

Lisa, thirty, diagnosed at twenty-three

Every little girl's dream,
taken away too soon.

What, no little child
with the same smile?

How can this be?
God, why did you take this from me?

To make me strong,
or to test me?

No, not me!
It cannot be!

While some days I'm weak
and just cannot speak

Other days I'm strong
knowing I can move on

Most days I keep hope alive
In knowing one day my childhood dream will arrive!

WHAT DO I SAY?

This first appeared as an exchange on the POFSG listserv.

Hi everybody!

Last month, Marta began a discussion on "What Do I Say?"—what to tell nosy relatives, friends, or whomever, about POF. Being recently diagnosed and just beginning to cope with all this condition signifies, I found the ensuing discussions very relevant and of great comfort.

Someone recently asked if anyone had saved the replies. I think I got most of them, if not all. I hope that I haven't distorted anyone's thoughts, and if I've disturbed the content and intent of those individuals' letters, I apologize.

I think these letters will help those who have recently joined our ranks and perhaps salve the souls of the "old timers." I appreciate the thoughtfulness, support and love these missives convey. Enjoy!

Love, Tina

Hello everyone!

I just went to a new doctor today and we have basically decided that I either don't have any eggs left, or if I do, science and my body have not figured out a way to grow them. I think I am finally accepting the diagnosis of POF. It has been a long year.

My question is:

Does anyone have any great comments they say whenever they are asked, "So, when are you going to start a family?"

I used to say, "Oh, maybe in a few years." I was just trying to put them off. Now, I want to say something to let them know that it is probably not possible, but I don't want to make them feel uncomfortable. I know some people say it is none of their business, but, I made a very good friend only because she told me she had her daughter through IVF. If she hadn't told me, I probably would never have contacted her and I would not have found such a great friend and supporter.

I want to say something that lets people know (but not too much). On the other hand, I want to say something that might make a connection with someone who needs some help.

Marta

About what to say when people ask... fortunately, I'm at the point where people have stopped asking! Yes, it does happen. However, when people did ask I finally reached the point where I had the strength to say, "I'm not able to have children." or "We're not able to have children." I finally realized there's no pussy-footing around that question! There's my two cents worth.

Pam

Funny you should ask how people are replying. Just this past weekend I ran into an old friend who has three children. After making small talk she asked the "question." My answer usually depends on what kind of day I'm having. My answer this day was, "Oh, I guess when I'm ready." Other times I have said, "Maybe in few years, I'm not really sure at this time." At other times I have said, "When everything starts working again." I have also been known to say simply, "I don't know."

It's definitely a very uncomfortable feeling when asked, and having to find the "right" answer without revealing your personal information. I get very angry at times! I wish people would think before they asked. Everyone who knows, or knew me, should know that I always wanted a

142

family, and if it were possible, I would probably have had children by now. Good luck!

Marlo

Here are some of my favorite options that I use:

Option #1 I tell people, "I have reproductive problems, but if the Lord steps in, I'll have more children."

Option #2 Sometimes I don't want to mention POF because I fear people will view me as elderly before my time, so I say I have ovarian problems. If the discussion goes further, I explain that for some unknown reason, my ovaries do not develop my eggs to full maturation, suitable for fertilization. I don't consider this far from the truth since they did find a maturing follicle on one ovary when I had my ultrasound at NIH. But I did not ovulate or have a period. I understand it is quite common for women with POF to have immature/undeveloped eggs instead of just being "out."

Option #3 Some consider this question ill mannered. Although I've never had the nerve, my dad says when folks ask rude questions to politely say, "If you'll forgive me for not answering, I'll forgive you for asking." Then move the conversation to another topic. He's the type who would say it. He believes if they are bold enough to ask such questions, they should be willing to hear bold answers and "get the message."

Helene

As far as people asking you about starting a family, I used to say, "Well, we're working on it." This was true before I was diagnosed with POF. Now, it feels like EVERYONE is wondering; when are they going to have kids, what's wrong with them? My friend asked me the other day and I told her the truth. I'm an open person and don't really mind. I said, "We were seeing a fertility specialist and it's just going to take awhile. I'm having all these tests done and it's probably going to involve some kind of medical intervention."

Personally, I don't care to lie or make up a little fib. Just tell them the general idea of it. You don't have to tell them all the details. This way, they'll also understand where you're coming from.

Valerie

RESOLVE, the national infertility support group, has a great section on what to say to the fertile world when asked about your plans. Their Website is www.resolve.org.

Janine

It mostly depends on you—whether you're comfortable revealing details about yourself. I've found that the best way to handle these inquiries is to be to the point and honest. The amount of detail I reveal depends on my relationship with the person. To a casual acquaintance I say, "I can't wait to have children, but I have infertility problems and need some help in order to do so." To friends and relatives I say, "I can't wait to have children. We have infertility problems and will do some IVF cycles in order to try to become pregnant."

My really close comrades get the whole story. I've found that by being so up front, you get more support. You may also help someone, too; By telling someone you are going through IVF they may know someone who is, too, and you could possibly benefit from an info exchange. I've made some close friendships by telling people I can't have children and they then confide that they've adopted, went through years of infertility, etc.

Bringing your infertility out of the closet can be very liberating. Plus, I think people should be told because it will perhaps educate the public about our situation. When people are educated, they're not so ignorant. Good luck!

Jennifer

I don't know exactly how to make a connection for others in similar situations when asked about a family. However, as far as the actual question of, "When are you going to start a family?" my answer was always, I have my husband and we are a family. This was primarily for the nosy aunts and cousins. We adopted a baby three years ago, and now all we hear is, "When will you be adopting you next baby?" It never ends!

Nicole

Make 'em feel guilty for prying. Cry a little and say that talking about it really makes you depressed. It used to be true for me!

Julie

I thought maybe I could shed the light of my own experience, since this is an issue I've dealt with for some twenty years now.

Infertility became an issue for me after I had been married for about three years the first time. I have a chronic illness that can be inherited; it isn't always, but there is a strong tendency for it to be. At the time, my doctors felt there was a distinct possibility that I could get pregnant, but would not be able to carry a baby to term without losing both the child and my own life. My health was in crisis at the time. I was five feet, four inches tall and weighed about sixty pounds. Because I have a digestive disease, I had had surgery to remove a good deal of my digestive tract, which is where most of our nutrients are absorbed. I was doing well to support my own body, much less a baby's and mine, too.

I tried BCP, but they made me deathly ill. This was in the days when they were much stronger than they are now, of course. I was so deathly ill from the combination of the BCP and my illness that the only option was a tubal ligation. Other methods of birth control were not feasible in my case, and I knew I could never handle the emotional aspect of making a decision to terminate a pregnancy if one occurred. So a tubal it was.

At the time I was dealing with the heartache of giving up my dream of having a family, every woman I knew seemed to be popping babies out like popcorn—especially those who didn't want them in the first place. I swear, some of them could just walk past a man and get pregnant. Only someone who really wants a child and can't have one knows how much pain that can bring.

People will inevitably ask questions. Some ask because they are concerned; they are happy with their families and want you to have the same joys—much like we all love people who are in love, because we know how great that is. Others ask to make small talk, but don't really want to know. It's just something to say. Others ask from pure nosiness; there's no getting around them. The rest can be stopped with the slightest indication that it's not a subject you want to talk about. You can give them an oblique answer such as, "When God sees fit to give us one," or, "We're practicing, but haven't had any luck yet." With any such answer they have sense enough not to push it. Those who really love you and care about you will be attuned to your discomfort in talking about it, if you are uncomfortable.

The nosy ones are a whole different group. They are like your basic bulldozers; they just keep coming long after they should. I'm with whoever said her father would tell them pointedly that it wasn't their business. When you get down to it, it's a very personal question to ask anyone. It's the equivalent of asking, "Is your hair really blonde? Is that a toupee? Are your teeth real?" What Dear Abby and Ann Landers would refer to as MYOB questions.

My offerings were along the lines of, "Why do you want to know?" or, "As soon as we decide to have a baby and have some news to tell, you will be among the first to know." Sometimes I would respond, "I'm sorry, but that question is a personal one that I don't feel the need to discuss with you."

The time may come when you have good news to share with the world. The time may come when you no longer have the burning desire to have a family of your own, and you realize that you can channel your love for children into so many other places where it is needed, as I have over time. Right now, I know this is very difficult for you to believe, as it was for me when I was where you are. I'm almost forty-six now, eight years into a new marriage and very happy with life as it is. I've learned along the way that there are always kids around to give your love to—far too many who desperately need it wherever they can get it. Even kids with parents and families need love from adults outside the family. I'm an "adopted" aunt to more kids than I can begin to count, and love every minute of it.

Do I have any regrets about having made the decision I did? No. Not any more. But it's taken me a long time to get here, and a lot of healing. You are fortunate to have many more options than I did, but I know I made the choice that was best for me at the time. I've made my peace with it. You have to, ultimately, whatever it is. With me, I knew that even if I adopted a child, someone else would have had to have taken care of it much of the time because of my health situation. I didn't want someone else being Mama to my baby. And I certainly didn't want to have to end a pregnancy. I don't judge those who do; I'm just saying I don't think I could have had the inner strength to deal with that.

I will tell you this. When it comes to anyone asking you about your "plans," that is no one's business but yours and your husband's. You can tell them as much or as little as you choose to, and they are the ones who must accept the answer. All you have to do is set the limit. As someone said earlier, it very often depends on the person, the day, and the attitude both you and they have. Whatever that is at any given time is fine. It's your life, and only you can judge what's enough information to dispense and what's over the line for you. Whatever that is, is fine.

The majority of you are very young still. You have options galore to explore before you give up on a family if you want one—everything from IVF, to adoption, to foster care, to volunteering to work with children in all sorts of areas. There are all kinds of things you can do. But as hard as it is to remember when your whole life seems to be centered around it, the ability to produce a child is only a very small part of who you are. Don't judge the whole package by the ribbon on top. Love it all. No matter what your destiny is as far as being a mother is concerned, there is a plan for your life or you wouldn't be here.

Don't you EVER allow anyone to demean you for not producing a child. Not everyone is meant to do that. And don't ever answer any questions, from anyone, that you aren't comfortable in answering. Trust your instinct. It's rarely wrong.

Angela

I have been reading all the comments concerning this topic. I must say, I agree with the ladies who have said go with your instinct. Having dealt with infertility issues for fifteen years now, I feel I have heard all the questions. What has worked best for me has been to be honest. I am not ashamed that I am not able to have children the "conventional way." Being infertile is only one aspect of who I am. Furthermore, infertility is who we are as a couple. This is as much my husbands "cross to bear" as it is mine. We have tried to meet it head-on, with dignity and grace. I found when I answered with a simple, "We are having difficulty conceiving," or "We would love to start now, but our bodies aren't cooperating," it always put the question back in the asker's lap. It also allows the asker to see that this is something you and your spouse are going through together. Those who are nosy never get the hint anyway. You have to be more direct, but never feel you have to apologize for your lack of fertility. You may have POF, but it doesn't have to have you. Those who truly care about you will want to know your hurts and pains; share with them. Infertility can rob you of many happy moments if you try to hide the pain or frustration. It will also rob you of joy if it consumes your every thought. There is a light at the end of the tunnel. It may not be the light you envisioned, but it is a light nonetheless. I live in a small community and I just assumed that everyone knew our two boys were adopted. I was off work so often because of surgeries and fertility procedures that I can't imagine anyone not knowing what we were going through, but it never ceases to amaze me when someone is surprised to find out that our boys are adopted or that we have had infertility problems. I think we get so caught up in the turmoil this puts in our lives that we just expect everyone to read it on our faces. Then when they do ask us a question we wonder how in the world they could be so insensitive. Give the asker the benefit of the doubt. If they are being idiots for asking, it doesn't matter how you answer. If they care, they want to know your hurts and pain. If they are just trying to make conversation, they will quickly change the subject once you tell them the truth. Don't let "The Question" add more stress to an already stressful situation. Answer it and move on.

Happy Life!
Rene

I just want to say "thanks." Thank you to all of you for your insights. Although they may have touched nerves this morning, I needed to hear that child-bearing is NOT everything I am, that I do still have a life. I tell this to myself time and time again, but you can never say it enough. Thank you for letting me hear it again.

Marta

POSTSCRIPT

This first appeared in Endless POFibilities—April 2001

Words of Wisdom, Thoughts from the Heart, by Jackie Curtis

Women on the POF message board were asked to share some words of wisdom. In one word, describe how you felt when you were first diagnosed? Now?

> Then: Devastated
> Now: Hopeful

> Then: Shocked
> Now: Accepting

> Then: Angry
> Now: Accepting

> Then: Devastated
> Now: Nothing can stand in my way

> Then: Couldn't believe
> Now: Still looking for a way of living with POF

> Then: Totally annihilated
> Now: Reluctant acceptance

What do you know now that you wish someone had told you when you were first diagnosed with POF?

> That POFers need continuous estrogen supplements and
> higher estrogen doses than menopausal women.

I wish someone would have told me my options (adoption, egg donor).

That I was not alone in my ordeal and that I was going to be all right!

That having POF did not have to run my life.

That my suspicion of having POF was correct and that they would have started investigative tests sooner.

"Tell me: What does it mean? How do you feel? Here is my shoulder if you need to cry, and here are my ears if you need to talk."

SOME FACTS ABOUT PREMATURE OVARIAN FAILURE

Premature ovarian failure (POF) is a loss of ovarian function in women under forty. Periods stop, estrogen levels are low and the follicle-stimulating hormone (FSH) level is elevated. Generally, it is said that the diagnosis requires at least four months without a period and two FSH tests, taken at least one month apart, that are greater than forty (some doctors will use thirty) mIU/ML.

Occasionally, women with POF experience spontaneous ovarian activity. If hormone tests are performed during those times, hormone levels could be in the normal range or only slightly out of range. This may lead to the elimination of POF as a diagnosis. Women who miss periods and have menopausal symptoms should have hormone testing repeated in one to two months.

POF is not menopause. Menopause occurs at an average age of fifty-one years and is a complete and irreversible cessation of menstrual activity. Most women with POF have intermittent ovarian function for many years. Unlike menopause, pregnancies are possible in women with POF.

The average age of onset is twenty-seven. It can occur as early as fourteen, before a girl has even had a period, to age thirty-nine. It occurs in approximately one percent of women.

Predictable menstrual cycles are the marker of healthy ovarian function during childbearing years. The ovary is both a reproductive organ and an endocrine gland. The two functions are tightly connected. A problem with the ovary results in problems with reproductive function and endocrine function.

POF is sometimes called premature menopause or early menopause. Use of appropriate terminology is important. Use of premature ovarian failure or ovarian insufficiency is preferred to premature menopause or early menopause.

There isn't a typical menstrual history for women with POF. Some women state that they feel as if they went to bed one night feeling fine and woke up the next morning with this problem. Some women start to miss periods, know they are not pregnant, but don't know the cause of the missed cycles. Some have normal periods, but develop hot flashes and can't figure out what is going on. In some women, the problem becomes apparent after they've had a baby and their periods never return. In others, it becomes apparent when they stop using birth control pills (BCP) and, again, their period never returns. Use of BCP may have hidden for years that a woman has POF, but there is no evidence that BCP can cause POF.

The most common symptoms, in addition to loss of periods or changes in periods, involve the loss of estrogen and include hot flashes, night sweats, irritability, dry skin, dry eyes, vaginal dryness, discomfort and pain during sexual intercourse, decreased libido, and decreased energy.

For most women a cause for their POF is never found. About twenty-five to thirty-five percent of women with POF have an associated autoimmune disorder. After autoimmunity, the most frequently identified cause is genetic. There are other reasons, such as a result of treatment for cancer with radiation or chemotherapy, or a hysterectomy with removal of the ovaries. In addition, infections have been associated with POF. A family history of POF is found in about four percent of the women.

Because the ovary is a source of hormones that help with other functions in the body in addition to pregnancy, most health care providers who are experts in POF say that all women with premature ovarian failure

Causes of Premature Ovarian Failure

Unknown (idiopathic)—For most women a cause is
   never found.
Autoimmune disease (these are some of the auto-
   immune diseases associated with POF)
      Thyroid dysfunction
      Polyglandular failure I and II
      Hypoparathyroidism
      Rheumatoid arthritis
      Idiopathic thrombocytopenia purpura (ITP)
      Diabetes
      Pernicious anemia
      Systemic lupus erythematosus—also called
      SLE or Lupus
      Addison's disease
Chromosomal/genetic
      Turner syndrome
      Androgen insensitivity syndrome (AIS)
Enzyme defects/metabolic abnormalities
      Galactosemia
Chemotherapy and radiation therapy related
Viral infection
Surgical
Inadequate gonadotropin (FSH and LH) secretion
   or action

should receive hormone replacement therapy (HRT) with estrogen and
progestin. HRT is given to relieve the symptoms of estrogen loss, to maintain bone density, and to reduce the risk of heart disease. A lack of estrogen at a young age may prevent women from achieving and maintaining
adequate bone density. There may be increased risk for osteoporosis and
bone fractures later in life. Low estrogen levels may also put women with
POF at higher risk for heart disease.

Estrogens can be taken in pill form, as a patch, or by oral contraceptives (OCP). Estrogen is generally taken every day. The choice depends on your own preference. It may take several different estrogens to find the one that is right for you. No studies have determined the appropriate dose to give women with POF. NIH investigators recommend doses that are double the amount of HRT given to women who are menopausal. The doses in OCP are more than is needed for relief of symptoms and bone maintenance. Some women prefer OCP to HRT because of the psychological impact of taking a menopause preparation versus something their friends are taking. The use of combination contraceptives provides appropriate doses of progestins.

Progestins must be taken in conjunction with estrogen. Estrogen without a progestin results in a continually stimulated uterine lining which greatly increases the risk of developing uterine cancer. When a progestin is taken with estrogen for ten to fourteen days per month in a cyclic fashion, the uterine lining builds up during the days when both hormones are taken. Wen the progestin is then stopped, the lining sheds and bleeding occurs for several days, much like a menstrual period. Some women prefer to take a continuous estrogen/progestin hormone regimen. In this case, women take a smaller dose of estrogen and progestin every day without varying the dose. The lower dose of the hormones results in the lining never becoming very thick, and because progestin is taken daily, there is never a withdrawal bleed. However, due to the high doses that women with POF take, this continuous HRT might not provide enough estrogen and progestin, and many doctors recommend, therefore, that hormones be taken cyclically.

HRT does not prevent ovulation and conception in women with POF. Women with POF have a five to ten percent chance of spontaneous pregnancy, so if bleeding fails to appear when expected, obtain a pregnancy test promptly. If a woman is taking HRT continuously, it may be more difficult to notice pregnancy signs. Even birth control pills may not suppress the rare spontaneous ovulations of women with POF.

If you are sexually active and do not want to become pregnant, you will need to use another form of birth control.

Women also produce small amounts of testosterone. Testosterone is often called the "male hormone." Women with POF have lower levels of testosterone compared to "normal" women their age. However, only a small percentage have levels below the lower limit of normal. Studies are underway to determine whether testosterone replacement should be a part of the standard therapy for POFers. Until results from these studies are available, testosterone replacement is considered for women who have persistent fatigue, low libido, and poor sense of well-being despite adequate estrogen replacement and when depression has been ruled out or adequately treated. Additionally, for women with both POF and Addison's disease, it is reasonable to offer testosterone replacement therapy, as these women cannot produce androgen.

No treatment has been proven to increase the ovulation rate or restore fertility in women with POF. Unproved treatments to restore fertility should be avoided because they have the potential of interfering with the development of a spontaneous pregnancy. Experimental treatment should be performed only under a review board-approved research protocol. The use of drugs such as Prednisone to restore ovarian function carries a risk of osteoporosis.

In addition to HRT, some tips for staying healthy are: take part in weight-bearing exercises for thirty minutes per day, at least three days per week, and consume 1,200 to 1,500 mg of calcium per day in your diet. If you aren't able to consume that much calcium, and most women don't, use elemental calcium supplementation. You also need to take vitamin D to supplement the calcium and have a DEXA bone test every two years.

Bone loss can occur if you go three months without a period. If you, your sister, another female relative or a friend skip your periods or have hot flashes, a doctor should be seen as soon as possible.

A diagnosis of POF can be devastating and depression can occur in women with POF. The NIH now recommends that women with POF receive three counseling sessions as part of routine POF care when they are diagnosed. Please ask for help, through the POF support group or counseling. We hope that this book will help on your path of healing and that you have found comfort here.

GLOSSARY

Addison's disease A rare endocrine or hormonal disorder that affects about one in 100,000 people. However, women with POF are three hundred times more likely than members of the general population to develop Addison's disease.

It occurs when the body's own immune system makes antibodies that attack and destroy the adrenal glands so the adrenal glands do not produce enough of the hormone cortisol. Cortisol's most important job is to help the body respond to stress. Additionally, it helps maintain blood pressure and cardiovascular function, slow the immune system's inflammatory response, balance the effects of insulin in breaking down sugar for energy, and regulate the metabolism of proteins, carbohydrates, and fats.

The symptoms of adrenal insufficiency usually begin gradually. It is characterized by weight loss, muscle weakness, fatigue, low blood pressure, and sometimes darkening of the skin in both exposed and unexposed parts of the body. Because of salt loss, craving of salty foods also is common.

In its early stages, adrenal insufficiency can be difficult to diagnose. Once diagnosed, it is easily treated with medication that replaces the hormones the adrenal glands are not making. However, if a person with untreated adrenal insufficiency experiences a stressful event, such as a severe illness, injury, or surgery, he or she can die from the condition.

AIS (androgen insensitivity syndrome) A condition that occurs when a fetus develops with a functioning Y chromosome, but an abnormality on the X chromosome that makes the developing baby completely or partially unable to respond to androgens. (Androgens are responsible for male secondary sexual characteristics—physical characteristics like beard growth and penis development.) As a result, the individual has non-functioning sex organs that do not produce sperm or eggs, no uterus, and all of the external physical characteristics of a female.

Atrophy A thinning of cells, tissues or organs. Here atrophy is used to describe "dry vagina," in which there is thinning of the vaginal walls that can lead to discomfort during intercourse and problems with sexual arousal. This occurs as a result of sustained low estrogen levels.

Beta-hCG A test to confirm or rule out pregnancy (also see hCG below).

Bone density test Sometimes called a bone mineral density test or bone density scan. It measures the strength and density of bones. It detects osteoporosis before a fracture occurs, predicts future fracture risk, and determines the rate of bone loss. When the test is repeated at a later point (generally, one to two years later) it can determine the rate of bone density change and monitor the effects of treatment.

Although there are different machines that measure bone density, most people today will get a bone density test from a machine using a technology called Dual Energy X-ray Absorptiometry—DEXA for short. All methods are painless, noninvasive, and safe.

Brain fog Refers to the short-term memory loss, confusion, and inability to concentrate that some women with POF experience. This issue is hotly debated in regards to menopausal women, with many medical researchers feeling that the problems are due to age, not menopause. However, the fact that many young women with POF experience similar problems lends credence to the argument that the problems are due to low estrogen. Far from being merely a hormone for the reproductive system, estrogen plays a role in many bodily functions. Some researchers suggest that the problems are due more to sleep impairment than to any direct effect of lack of estrogen in the brain. Sleep impairment is a common problem with POF, due to night sweats.

Clomid A drug that fools the brain into thinking estrogen levels are too low. In response, the pituitary gland in the brain secretes more FSH to stimulate the ovary to produce more estrogen and to develop one or more eggs.

Corpus luteum The yellow gland formed by ruptured follicles after ovulation. The corpus luteum produces progesterone and, in the event of fertilization, provides the required progesterone to support early pregnancy until the placenta is formed. The corpus luteum also produces some estrogen. In the absence of fertilization, the lifespan of the corpus luteum is approximately fourteen days.

DE (donor egg) Donor egg programs allow women who are unable to produce their own eggs for fertilization to utilize the eggs of another woman. Via ovarian stimulation and *in vitro* fertilization (IVF) eggs are retrieved from another women, fertilized by a man's sperm and the resulting embryos are implanted in the recipient's uterus. The woman donating the eggs goes through preparations necessary to retrieve multiple fertile eggs by taking drugs such as Lupron, Gonal-F, and hCG. The eggs are retrieved in a surgical procedure. The recipient takes hormonal preparations to make her uterus ready to accept embryos for implantation.

In the United States, women typically receive financial compensation for donating eggs, meaning that eggs are readily available, though not plentiful. In some other English speaking countries, like Canada and the United Kingdom, women do not receive financial compensation, and therefore eggs tend to be more difficult to obtain. In the United States, some insurance companies cover at least part of the costs of these procedures. The total cost may be $15,000 or more.

Endocrinologist A physician who specializes in the diagnosis and treatment of conditions affecting the endocrine system such as diabetes and thyroid problems.

Endometriosis A painful condition resulting from endometrial (uterine lining) tissue being abnormally located outside the uterus, usually in the pelvis and abdomen. Pain is caused when the endometrial tissue bleeds during menstrual periods, resulting in local irritation and scarring.

Estradiol (E2) One of the three major estrogen hormones which women produce. The other two are estrone and estriol. Estradiol is the most abundant type of estrogen found in women during their fertile years, and it is also the most powerful. The ovarian follicle produces it as it develops during the first half of the menstrual cycle and it is excreted by the corpus luteum after ovulation.

Estradiol is responsible for development of the secondary sexual characteristics and maturation of long bones.

Estrogen One of a group of hormones, including estriol, estrone, and estradiol, that control and maintain the female reproductive system. Estrogens and other hormones, especially progesterone, are involved in the menstrual cycle and pregnancy. The main source of estrogen in normally cycling women is the ovarian follicle.

FET (frozen embryo transfer) Unused frozen embryos from a previous IVF cycle are thawed and transferred to the recipient's uterus in a subsequent IVF cycle.

Freehold house A British term defining a house on which the mortgage has been paid off.

FSH (follicle stimulating hormone) A hormone that is produced by the pituitary gland that stimulates growth of follicles in the ovaries and the production of estrogen. FSH levels can be determined by a blood test. A continually high FSH level can be an indicator of POF. High FSH levels are used in diagnosis of POF. High FSH levels mean that the body is trying very hard to encourage the ovaries to work.

Gonal-F A chemically synthesized hormone that is similar to FSH. It is used in the treatment of certain types of infertility to directly stimulate the ovaries to produce multiple eggs. It is also used by the donor in an egg donor program. Gonal-F is administered just under the skin using a small needle. Gonal-F is not effective for women with POF because women with POF already have very high levels of FSH, and their ovaries are not responding to it adequately. Giving additional FSH in the form of Gonal-F will therefore not have any significant effect on fertility.

GP (general practitioner) A physician who provides and coordinates primary, and continuing, comprehensive health care to individuals and families.

hCG (human chorionic gonadotropin) A hormone produced in large amounts in pregnancy and is the basis for pregnancy tests. hCG also occupies the LH receptor on the ovary and serves the same function as LH, only it's longer-acting. For this reason, hCG is the drug of choice for inducing the final stages of follicle maturation and ovulation (which is normally done by LH in a regularly cycling woman), and is given as a single injection for this purpose.

Hormone replacement therapy (HRT) Replacement of female hormones (estrogen, progestin, and sometimes testosterone) the body no longer produces. People commonly associate its use with woman who are postmenopausal. However, women who are diagnosed with POF are also generally prescribed HRT as well. The therapy is widely, but not universally, thought to help prevent osteoporosis and heart disease and minimize the symptoms often associated with hormonal imbalance, such as hot flashes, vaginal dryness and atrophy, mood swings and night sweats.

Some have suggested that the term HRT is more applicable to women with POF since they need to replace the hormones that are not being produced by the ovary. Older women in menopause actually receive hormone extension therapy. Recent research has questioned the benefit of HRT in postmenopausal women as it has been shown to increase the risk of breast and uterine cancer and is linked to an increased risk of blood clots and stroke. The extent that these findings apply to POFers, if at all, is questionable, as the studies were conducted in older women who received HRT past the time their ovaries naturally stopped producing the hormones.

Hot flashes/hot flushes A sudden, temporary feeling of warmth often through the face, neck and chest experienced by most women during menopause and POF. They are the most common early symptom when blood levels of estrogen decrease. In the UK, the term "flush" is used in place of "flash."

Hymen A fold of mucous membrane that partly covers the entrance to the vagina and is usually ruptured when sexual intercourse takes place for the first time. However, the hymen is fragile and can be broken in many different ways, including through intense sports or tampon use.

Hypothyroid (hypothyroidism) An autoimmune disease of the thyroid gland which prevents it from producing adequate amounts of thyroid hormone. Symptoms include feeling cold, exhaustion, fertility problems, menstrual changes, weight changes, and dry, brittle nails. The missing hormone is replaced by thyroid hormone replacement drugs.

Hysterosalpingogram (HSG) An x-ray procedure performed to determine if the fallopian tubes are open and to see the shape of the uterine cavity. It involves an injection of dye through the cervix into the uterus.

ICSI (intracytoplasmic sperm injection) Direct injection of a single sperm into an egg. This IVF technique is usually used for couples when the male partner has a very low sperm count.

IVF (*in vitro* fertilization) A procedure which involves using hormone drugs to stimulate egg production, removing a ripened egg, or eggs from a female's ovary, fertilizing it with sperm, incubating the dividing cells in a laboratory dish (hence the term "test tube baby") and then replacing the developing embryo(s) in the uterus at the appropriate time through the cervix.

Luteinizing hormone (LH) A female hormone produced by the pituitary that in females regulates ovulation and menstruation. LH increases near the middle of the menstrual cycle and causes the maturation of the egg. Ovulation occurs approximately twenty-four to thirty-six hours after the LH surge.

Lupron A drug that inhibits the release of LH and FSH from the pituitary and "shuts down" a woman's natural hormone cycle.

Melasma An area of tan or brown patches that usually appears on the face. The pigmented area often appears like a mask across the cheeks and forehead or on the upper lip. These patches do not itch and are not red or swollen.

Melasma results from increased skin pigmentation, the cause of which is presently unknown. However, the relationship of melasma to BCP and HRT use suggests hormones are a potential cause, at least in some cases.

Menopause Refers to the normal cessation of periods. The average age of menopause for American women is fifty-one. It is actually a process, not a specific moment. For several years preceding the complete cessation of menses, a woman might experience an irregularity of menses, and menopausal symptoms that occur more at some times of the month than others. During the time period when these symptoms begin, the woman is considered to be perimenopausal. If she has not experienced menstruation in more than a year, then she is considered to be menopausal.

NIH (National Institutes of Health) The Federal focal point for medical research in the United States. The goal of NIH research is to acquire new knowledge to help prevent, detect, diagnose, and treat disease and disability, from the rarest genetic disorder to the common cold. The NICHD (National Institute of Child Health and Human Development), one of NIH's twenty-seven institutes and centers, conducts clinical research on POF. NIH is one of eight health agencies of the Public Health Service that, in turn, is part of the U.S. Department of Health and Human Services. The main campus is located outside Washington, DC.

Ob/Gyn (obstetrician-gynecologist) A physician who specializes in the management of pregnancy and diseases affecting the female reproductive system.

Osteoporosis A condition resulting in weakened bones and, eventually, bone loss. It is caused by poor absorption of calcium and other minerals into the bones, resulting from persistently low levels of estrogen and testosterone. Estrogen and, to a certain extent, testosterone is important in building and maintaining bone strength.

Ovral A brand name for a birth control pill (BCP). It is known as a monophasic contraceptive, as all pills in the pack contain the same amounts of hormones. It is also a combination oral contraceptive as it contains both estrogen and progestin. Combination BCPs inhibit ovulation in women with normally functioning ovaries by suppressing FSH and LH. They also cause alterations in the cervical mucus and the endometrium to reduce the likelihood of implantation of a fertilized egg. May be taken by women with POF as their HRT. However, birth control pills may not suppress the rare spontaneous ovulations of women with POF. If you are sexually active and do not want to become pregnant, you will need to use another form of birth control.

Pergonal The gonadotropins, luteinizing and follicle-stimulating hormones, recovered from the urine of postmenopausal women that are used to stimulate the ovaries to produce multiple eggs in various fertility treatments.

Progesterone A hormone produced by the body that most noticeably has the effect of thickening the lining of the uterus to ready it for implantation by an egg. It is usually produced by the corpus luteum; that is, the cyst in the ovary that remains after an egg is released. Used, along with estrogen, in HRT.

RE (reproductive endocrinologist) A physician with advanced training in the specialty of endocrinology (hormones) and infertility in addition to training in obstetrics and gynecology. An RE typically treats infertility, and may also treat problems related to menopause, and hormonal disorders in women such as premature ovarian failure.

Withdrawal bleed When HRT is taken cyclically, progesterone causes the lining of the uterus to shed and causes a regular bleed similar to a light period. The withdrawal bleed happens after the progesterone part is stopped. However, these are not "true" periods as HRT does not cause ovulation or restore fertility.

WHERE TO FIND HELP

Following is a list* of organizations, publications and Websites recommended by members of the POFSG. Only resources that POFers suggested are included. We hope some of these will be useful to you. Be advised that some of the groups listed have little funding and often rely on volunteers. Addresses and phone numbers may change if coordinators relocate. The information is current as of our printing. If readers become aware of outdated or updated information, please contact the POFSG at FACESOFPOF@pofsupport.org or 703 913-4787.

POF/Premature Menopause**

Organizations

The Daisy Network
PO Box 183
Rossendale
BB4 6WZ
United Kingdom
membership&media@daisynetwork.org.uk
www.daisynetwork.org.uk

The Daisy Network Premature Menopause Support Group is the only UK group for women with this condition. It is a registered charity run by women who have had a premature menopause and provides

---

* Several entries cross organizations/publications/Websites within the resource section. We have included the resource only one time. For example, The Premature Menopause Book, is listed under publications, but there is a Website connected with it. These are grouped together.

** The term, "Premature Menopause," although inaccurate, has been used extensively by medical personnel and lay people, and so is included. It is also the term used in the U.K.

advice and support. The Daisy Network allows members to share information about their personal experience of POF, provides a support network of people you can talk to, and provides information on treatments and research within the fields of HRT and assisted conception.

The International Premature Ovarian Failure Support Group, Inc. (POFSG)
PO Box 23643
Alexandria, VA 22304
703 913-4787
info@pofsupport.org
www.POFSupport.org

The mission of the POFSG is to provide community, support, and information to women with Premature Ovarian Failure (POF) and their loved ones; to increase public awareness and understanding of POF; and to work with health care professionals to better understand this condition.

A nonprofit organization, it provides information and support for women, friends and family members dealing with POF. The group offers message boards, listserv, Dr. Answer Line, quarterly newsletters, FAQ and annual conferences.

North American Menopause Society (NAMS)
PO Box 94527
Cleveland, OH 44101
440 442-7550
Fax: 440 442-2660
info@menopause.org
www.menopause.org

NAMS is a nonprofit organization dedicated to promoting women's health during mid-life and beyond through an understanding of menopause. Although membership is limited to professionals, they provide information on perimenopause, early menopause, menopause symptoms, long-term health effects of estrogen loss and a wide variety of therapies to enhance health to the general public.

Publications

Davis, Susan R., *Our Health, Our Lives* (Australia: Allen & Unwin, 1997).

This book presents a balanced appraisal of women's health issues ranging from risk factors for breast cancer and lifestyle prevention strategies to natural therapies for a variety of problems. Includes a chapter on POF.

Domar, Alice D. and Dreher, Henry, *Healing Mind, Healthy Woman* (Delta, 1997).

This book uses the mind-body connection to help control stress associated with infertility and menopause, as well as other women's health issues. This book helps to focus on what you can do to improve your overall health. Audiotapes are available as an adjunct to the book.

Lee, John R. and Hopkins, Virginia, *What your Doctor May Not Tell You About Menopause: The Breakthrough Book on Natural Progesterone* (Warner Books, 1996).

This book covers the benefits of natural progesterone, the history and politics of the medical and drug establishment, the biochemistry and dynamics of hormones and how they get out of balance, and how to prevent hormone imbalance and stay healthy. Geared to women in menopause.

Nelson, Lawrence M., M.D., MBA, *Spontaneous Premature Ovarian Failure: Young Women, Special Needs* (Menopause Management, July/August 2001).

Written in a medical journal, this article nonetheless is excellent reading for women with POF. Thorough discussion of all aspects of POF. Give a copy to your health care provider.

Petras, Kathryn, *The Premature Menopause Book: When the "Change of Life" Comes too Early* (Quill, 1999).

Written by a woman with premature menopause. This book covers health and emotional issues, HRT options and natural supplements, lists resources, Websites and support groups, and includes interviews from women in their twenties and thirties coping with this situation.

There is also a Website based on the book at: www.early-menopause.com. In addition to excerpts from the book, it includes information not in the book, such as continually updated information on the current forms of HRT available, news items, special articles on osteoporosis, hormone testing, birth control pills and a variety of other issues.

Singer, Dani, *Premature Menopause: A Multidisciplinary Approach* (Taylor and Francis, 2000).

Although written for health professionals, women with some knowledge of POF will get much out of it. The editors bring together experts from a range of disciplines including endocrinology, gynecology, general practice, nursing, psychotherapy, complementary medicine and clinical psychology, as well as hearing from women themselves. Offers up-to-date information on the topic, as well as practical suggestions for improved health care. Catherine Corp, POFSG founder, contributed to the chapter, Self-help and support groups.

Vliet, Elizabeth Lee, *Screaming to be Heard: Hormone Connections Women Suspect and Doctors Ignore* (M Evans & Co., 2nd edition 2001).

Vliet convincingly defends hormone replacement therapy, although controversial, as a corrective and preventive treatment, providing it is individualized and integrated with alternative therapies. Aimed at health care professionals and informed lay readers.

Vliet, Elizabeth Lee, *It's My Ovaries, Stupid!* (Scribner, 2003).

This book offers a serious and comprehensive look at hormone dysfunction in women of all ages.

Vliet provides a complete guide to ovaries, explaining how they work and what happens when they don't work properly, along with surgical and other treatment. Included are questionnaires so readers can self-diagnose and prepare themselves before visiting a doctor.

Vliet, Elizabeth Lee, *Women, Weight and Hormones* (M Evans & Co., 2001).

The author explains how estrogen and progesterone levels change and interact at mid-life to slow female metabolism, which may lead to weight gain. Through a combination of hormonal balance, healthy eating, exercise and improved self-esteem she states the pattern can be reversed. The cornerstone of her book is the "meal action plan" (MAP).

Connected with these books is:
HER Place®: Health Enhancement and Renewal for Women, Inc.
PO Box 64507
Tucson, AZ 85728
520 797-9131
Fax: 520 797-2948
HerPlace4U@aol.com
www.herplace.com

A women's health center located in Tucson, Arizona, the center offers a host of services focusing on the integration of hormonal changes with physical, emotional and social aspects of women's lives. The author is the founder and Medical Director for HER Place®.

Websites

Center for Young Women's Health, Children's Hospital
333 Longwood Avenue, 5th floor
Boston, MA 02115
617 355-2994
Fax: 617 232-3136
cywh@tch.harvard.edu
www.youngwomenshealth.org/pof.html

Recognizing the urgent need for education, clinical care, research, and health care advocacy for adolescent girls and young women, Children's Hospital of Boston has created an initiative, the Center for Young Women's Health. International in scope and collaborative in nature, they are committed to improving the health and well-being of adolescent girls. They invite you to learn about their research projects and health care provider education, explore their clinical services, and visit their Resource Center. Publication: *Premature Ovarian Failure: A Guide for Teens* is available on their Website.

Project AWARE (Association of Women for the Advancement of Research and Education)

www.project-aware.org

A Website by women, for women offering objective and comprehensive health information, especially related to menopause, perimenopause, and postmenopause.

Adoption

Organizations

National Adoption Center
1500 Walnut Street, Suite 701
Philadelphia, PA 19102
800 TO-ADOPT (800 862-3678)
nac@nationaladoptioncenter.org
www.adopt.org
   The National Adoption Center expands adoption opportunities for children throughout the United States, particularly for children with special needs and those from minority cultures.

National Adoption Information Clearinghouse
330 C Street, SW
Washington, DC 20447
703 352-3488 or 888 251-0075
Fax: 703 385-3206
naic@calib.com
www.calib.com/naic
   A comprehensive resource on all aspects of adoption. Maintained by the U.S. Department of Health and Human Services Administration for Children and Families.

U.S. Department of State
Bureau of Consular Affairs
Overseas Citizens Services
Office of Children Issues
SA-29, 4th Floor
U.S. Department of State
Washington, DC 20520

888 407-4747 (8 a.m. to 8 p.m.)
Fax: 202 736-9133
http://travel.state.gov/adopt

The Office of Children Issues coordinates policy and provides information on international adoption to the public. Because adoption is a private legal matter within the judicial sovereignty of the nation where the child resides, the Department of State cannot intervene on behalf of an individual U.S. citizen in foreign courts. They offer general information and assistance regarding the adoption process in over 60 countries.

Publications

Adoptive Families Magazine
42 West 38th St., Suite 901
New York, NY 10018
800 372-3300
Fax: 646 366-0842
letters@adoptivefam.com
www.adoptivefamilies.com

Adopting is a special act that requires a great deal of information both before and after the adoption. Adoptive Families fills this need in a thorough and sensitive manner. Articles include legal issues, psychology, practical activities and methods for enhancing adoptive family life. Personal experiences of other adoptive parents serve as clear models, and reviews of books and other media keep parents current.

Hicks, Randall B., *Adopting in America: How to Adopt in One Year* (SCB Distributors, 2nd edition February 1999).

This book clearly explains all the ways to adopt, pros and cons for each, and describes the processes. It also contains state-by-state descriptions of adoption laws and recommendations for adoption resources in each state.

Johnston, Patricia Irwin, *Adopting after Infertility* (Indiana: Perspectives Press, 1996).

Information about all the losses you are experiencing, how to decide on possible solutions with your partner and all the aspects that involve choosing adoption.

Wadia-Ells, Susan, *The Adoption Reader: Birth Mothers, Adoptive Mothers, and Adopted Daughters Tell Their Stories* (Seal Press, 1995).

Essays written by birth mothers, adoptive mothers, and adopted daughters. This book evokes strong emotions that people going through an adoption will experience.

Websites

www.adoption.about.com

Comprehensive collection of online resources about adoption and adoption issues.

www.adoptionforums.com

Adoption-related message board. Covers many topics including international and domestic adoption issues.

Donor egg/Surrogacy

Websites

Looking To Be A Mom Through Egg Donation

www.network54.com/Hide/Forum/57451

Interactive forum for those considering or undergoing IVF with donor egg and need emotional support.

Mothers Via Egg Donation Listserv and Online Support Group

TASC@surrogacy.com

www.surrogacy.com/online_support/mved

A forum open only to women who have been, or are attempting to become, mothers through egg donation or surrogacy. Because this is a closed area, members can communicate freely and openly with each other without the worry of unwanted visitors.

Surrogate Mothers Online

Info@surromomsonline.com

www.surromomsonline.com

Online resource and virtual meeting ground for surrogates and intended parents.

Fertility/Infertility

Organizations

InterNational Council on Infertility Information Dissemination, Inc. (INCIID)
PO Box 6836
Arlington, VA 22206
703 379-9178
www.inciid.org

INCIID (pronounced "inside") is a nonprofit organization committed to providing the most current information regarding the diagnosis, treatment, and prevention of infertility and pregnancy loss.

RESOLVE: The National Infertility Association
1310 Broadway
Somerville, MA 02144
HelpLine number: 888 623-0744
Office: 617 623-1156
info@resolve.org
www.resolve.org

RESOLVE is a national organization that provides timely, compassionate support and information, through advocacy and public education, to individuals who are experiencing infertility issues.

Publications

Weschler, Toni, *Taking Charge of Your Fertility: The Definitive Guide to Natural Birth Control, Pregnancy Achievement, and Reproductive Health* (Quill; Revised edition, November 2001).
www.TCOYF.com

This book explains what "normal" reproductive cycles are supposed to be like for women, and what signs to look for that you may be having problems. For women with POF, it is helpful to know what should be happening and how to know if our bodies suddenly decide to start acting normal again!

Schalesky, Marlo, *Empty Womb, Aching Heart — Hope and Help for Those Struggling With Infertility* (Minnesota: Bethany House Publishers, 2001).

This book is a collection of short stories, based on the experiences of real men and women who struggle with infertility. Each story explores a slightly different aspect of infertility, but all have a strong Christian foundation.

Those in the middle of the infertility journey will find these stories encouraging and comforting for several reasons. First, they help you to realize that you are neither alone nor crazy—your experience is just the same as many others. Second, this books avoids the all-too-common "and then we had a baby!" happy ending. While all the stories end on a hopeful note, more often than not it is because the characters learn new ways to cope, or rely on God for comfort. Finally, both men's and women's perspectives on infertility are addressed.

Websites

About Infertility
www.infertility.about.com

Comprehensive collection of online resources about infertility and infertility related issues.

Child of My Dreams
www.childofmydreams.com

Provides online information and advice for people facing the challenges of infertility and adoption.

Conceiving Concepts Inc.
www.conceivingconcepts.com

A fertility products and services company. An advocate for those struggling with fertility problems. Their goal is to arm you with the tools and information to help you on your pathway to parenthood, from fertility products to a safe place to meet people who understand.

Fertile Thoughts
www.fertilethoughts.net

Help and support for infertile couples going through medical treatment of infertility, adoption as well as to support woman going through surrogacy. Provides information from finding the perfect doctor, to your diagnosis, to treatment and options to insurance issues. They also provide resources and links to childrearing material.

Hope For Fertility
www.HopeForFertility.com

A support group for the emotional needs of those challenged by fertility issues. Hope continues to pick up where most doctors leave off, by providing the type of support that only one fertility patient can offer another through understanding. Support is given through chat room, message boards, Hope SurvivalGuide, and Guardian Angel Program.

Infertility Resources
www.ihr.com/infertility

Provides extensive infertility information including IVF, ICSI, infertility clinics, donor egg and surrogacy programs, natural infertility treatment, male infertility doctors, sperm banks, pharmacies, infertility products, sperm testing, infertility support, and drug and medication information.

www.ihr.com/infertility/articles/ovumdonation.html is the online resource for information about egg donations and egg donors.

IVF Connections
www.ivfconnections.com

Connects people going through IVF to information, support, and others going through the same experiences. IVF Connections features IVF bulletin boards, IVF email lists, IVF chatrooms, IVF questions and answers, IVF stories, IVF links and an IVF in Canada section.

Shared Journey

sharedjourney@sharedjourney.com
www.sharedjourney.com

Dedicated to providing quality information on topics such as infertility, miscarriage, surrogacy, pregnancy after infertility, living child-free, and adoption. Information is supplied by well known reproductive endocrinologists, psychologists, adoption professionals and links through various sites.

Nutrition

Publications

Ricciotti, Hope and Connelly, Vincent, *The Menopause Cookbook — How to Eat Now and for the Rest of Your Life*. Add estrogen to your diet naturally (W.W. Norton & Company, Inc., 2000). As a gynecologist, Dr. Ricciotti counsels women on the best way to stay healthy and lower the impact of the side effects of menopause. In *The Menopause Cookbook*, she gives a brief guide to the changes of menopause and your body's new nutritional needs. Whether you have decided for or against hormone replacement therapy, Dr. Ricciotti recommends adding phytoestrogens as well as calcium and antioxidants to your diet. Eating plenty of foods high in natural estrogen, calcium, and fiber will help keep you healthy and feeling great, while reducing the potential side effects of the menopausal years, from hot flashes to osteoporosis.

Simopoulos, Artemis P. and Robinson, Jo, *The Omega Diet: The Lifesaving Nutritional Program Based on the Diet of the Island of Crete* (HarperCollins Publishers, 1999). *The Omega Diet* is a natural, time-tested diet that balances the essential fatty acids in your diet. It is packed with delicious foods that contain "good" fats, including real salad dressing, cheese, eggs, fish—even the occasional chocolate dessert—and an abundance of antioxidant-rich fruits, vegetables, and legumes. *The Omega Diet* provides: seven simple dietary guidelines for optimal physical and mental health, a concise guide to the foods you need to restore your body's nutritional balance, a diet plan that lets you eat fat as you lose fat, fifty delicious recipes that are quick and easy to prepare, and a comprehensive three-week menu to help you get started.

General Women's Health

Organizations

National Women's Health Resource Center, Inc. (NWHRC)
120 Albany Street, Suite 820
New Brunswick, NJ 08901
877 986-9472
Fax: 732 249-4671
vngethe@healthywomen.org
www.healthywomen.org

The national clearinghouse for women's health information and resources. The information provided is comprehensive, objective, and supported by an advisory council comprised of the nation's leading medical and health experts.

Publications

Northrup, Christiane, M.D., *Women's Bodies, Women's Wisdom* (Bantam Books; Revised and Updated edition, March 1998)

This guide goes far beyond standard self-help books, assessing women's health within the context of their work, families and society. The author, a holistic physician specializing in obstetrics and gynecology, seeks to illuminate the basic conditions of women's lives that lead to their health problems.

Websites

Holistic online
http://holisticonline.com

Comprehensive information about health. Features conventional, alternative, integrative, and mind-body medicine.

JAMA & Archives Journals

http://pubs.ama-assn.org

Register as a guest for access to selected free content to the Journal of the American Medical Association (JAMA) and Archives Journals from January 1998 forward.

Medscape Ob/Gyn & Women's Health

www.medscape.com/womenshealthhome

Medscape is organized by medical specialty. Each specialty has its own Website. Specialty content is evaluated, created, and presented under the guidance of editorial and scientific advisory boards. This is a general site about women's health, infertility, and POF. Full text medical journals are available for download. Although this site is directed at clinicians and other healthcare professionals, you'll find perhaps the most comprehensive access to medicine on the Internet.

Research

National Institutes of Health (NIH), Section on Women's Health, POF Studies

9000 Rockville Pike

Bethesda, MD 20892

Contact: Vien Vanderhoof, R.N., C.R.N.P., at 877 206-0911 to obtain information about enrollment in the studies.

www.nih.gov

The Website contains articles and information about current POF research studies. A twenty-one page pamphlet, *Do I have Premature Ovarian Failure?*, was published in August 2003.

Special POF concerns

Androgen Insensitivity Syndrome

Website

Androgen Insensitivity Syndrome Support Group (AISSG)

AISSG USA
PO Box 2148
Duncan, OK 73534-2148
aissgusa@hotmail.com

AISSG Canada
(East)
#206, 115 The Esplanade
Toronto, Ontario
M5E 1Y7
sallie@ican.net
(West)
#17, 3031 Williams Road
Richmond, B.C.
V7E 1H9
lesnick@shaw.ca

AISSG UK
PO Box 269, Banbury
Oxon, OX15 6YT
email: orchids@talk21.com
www.medhelp.org/www/ais

AISSG is a peer support organization. Their goal is to help people who have AIS, have good reason to believe they, or a family member has AIS or a closely related biological intersex condition; and clinicians.

Hysterectomy

Website

Hyster Sisters
2436 S. I-35 E. Suite 376-184
Denton, TX 76205-4900
www.hystersisters.com

Hystersisters.com is a woman to woman support Website for hysterectomy recovery. It is neither anti nor pro hysterectomy. Rather, it is an online community of women who give and receive support for hysterectomy decisions and recovery. Hystersisters.com offers resources and kindness so that visitors can discover options and make decisions for themselves.

CONTACTING US

If you are interested in communicating with any of the authors, most are open to talking with others about POF. Please contact us by phone or e-mail to be put in touch with a contributor.

We would like to hear your reactions to the stories in this collection. Please let us know your favorites and how they affected you.

Also, please send us your stories you would like to see published in future editions of *Faces of POF* or *POFibilities*, the POFSG quarterly newsletter. To obtain a copy of our submissions guidelines, please email or check our Website.

Faces of POF
POFSG
PO Box 23643
Alexandria, VA 22304
703 913-4787
FACESOFPOF@POFSupport.org
www.pofsupport.org

Order *Faces of POF* for a Friend

Telephone orders: 1-888-616-7720
Fax orders: 1-970-221-4884
E-mail orders: books@northfortynews.com
Postal orders: Ink & Scribe
3101 Kintzley Court, Unit J
LaPorte, CO   80535-9393

Please send me:

_____ copies of *Faces of POF* @ $16.99 per copy

Subtotal _____

Sales tax:

Please add 3.7% for products shipped to Colorado addresses

Subtotal _____

Shipping:

US: $3.00 for the first book and $1.50 for each additional book

Subtotal _____

International: Call for prices   _____

TOTAL   _____

Payment: __ Check

__ Credit Card: __ Visa __ MasterCard

Credit card orders will be billed by Wise River Companies, Inc.

Card Number: _____

Name on card: _____

Exp. date: _____ / _____

Signature: _____

Shipping address:

Name: _____

Address: _____

City: _____ State: ____ Zip: _____

Telephone: _____

E-mail address: _____

Order *Faces of POF* for a Friend

Telephone orders: 1-888-616-7720
Fax orders: 1-970-221-4884
E-mail orders: books@northfortynews.com

Postal orders: Ink & Scribe
     3101 Kintzley Court, Unit J
     LaPorte, CO   80535-9393

Please send me:

_____ copies of *Faces of POF* @ $16.99 per copy

        Subtotal _____

Sales tax:

     Please add 3.7% for products shipped to Colorado addresses

        Subtotal _____

Shipping:

     US: $3.00 for the first book and $1.50 for each additional book

        Subtotal _____

     International: Call for prices _____

     TOTAL _____

Payment: __ Check

        __ Credit Card: __ Visa __ MasterCard

Credit card orders will be billed by Wise River Companies, Inc.

Card Number: _____

Name on card: _____

Exp. date: _____ / _____

Signature: _____

Shipping address:

Name: _____

Address: _____

City: _____ State: ___ Zip: _____

Telephone: _____

E-mail address: _____